super simple
KETO

SIX INGREDIENTS OR LESS TO TURN YOUR GUT INTO A FAT-BURNING MACHINE

AIMEE ARISTOTELOUS & RICHARD OLIVA

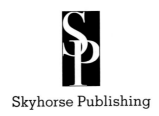

Skyhorse Publishing

Skyhorse Publishing books may be purchased in bulk at special discounts for sales promotion, corporate gifts, fund-raising, or educational purposes. Special editions can also be created to specifications. For details, contact the Special Sales Department, Skyhorse Publishing, 307 West 36th Street, 11th Floor, New York, NY 10018 or info@skyhorsepublishing.com.

Skyhorse® and Skyhorse Publishing® are registered trademarks of Skyhorse Publishing, Inc.®, a Delaware corporation.

Visit our website at www.skyhorsepublishing.com.

10 9 8 7 6 5 4 3 2 1

Library of Congress Cataloging-in-Publication Data
Names: Aristotelous, Aimee, author. | Oliva, Richard, author.
Title: *Super simple keto*: six ingredients or less to turn your gut into a
   fat-burning machine / Aimee Aristotelous and Richard Oliva.
Description: New York, NY: Skyhorse Publishing, [2021] | Includes
   bibliographical references and index. | Identifiers: LCCN 2021018322 (print) |
LCCN 2021018323 (ebook) | ISBN
   9781510765481 (hardcover) | ISBN 9781510765498 (ebook)
Subjects: LCSH: Ketogenic diet. | Low-carbohydrate diet—Recipes. |
   Reducing diets—Recipes. | Weight loss. | LCGFT: Cookbooks.
Classification: LCC RC374.K46 A756 2021 (print) | LCC RC374.K46 (ebook) |
   DDC 641.5/6383--dc23
LC record available at https://lccn.loc.gov/2021018322
LC ebook record available at https://lccn.loc.gov/2021018323

Cover design by Daniel Brount
Cover image from iStockphoto

Print ISBN: 978-1-5107-6548-1
Ebook ISBN: 978-1-5107-6549-8

Printed in China

Dedicated to those who want to reach their wellness goals,
without spending hours in the kitchen.

Contents

Introduction

Hello! Welcome to *Super Simple Keto*. Before you read any further, the following three pages will help you gauge if this book is right for you, and your health and weight loss goals. We are sure you have heard of the ketogenic diet before but you may not be familiar with exactly what it entails. This introduction serves as a snap summary and analysis so you can quickly get acquainted with the protocol to decide if it's one you can see yourself having success with. First of all, below you will find three examples of standard *Super Simple Keto* meals which make up a typical one-day plan. They consist of many regular whole foods that are moderately inexpensive and can be found in most mainstream grocery stores. If you can see yourself eating these meals, continue on.

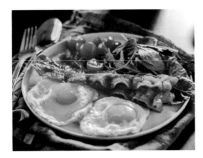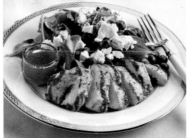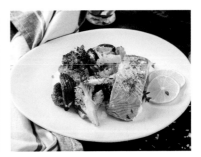

Simply put, for keto, you just need (roughly) 75 percent fat, 20 percent protein, and five percent carbohydrates. People safely lose as much as fifteen to twenty pounds per month just following this super simple protocol. That's why the ketogenic (or keto) diet is the most talked about nutrition plan of this past decade.

If the following grocery list contains at least 50 percent of the foods you eat (or wouldn't mind eating) on a normal basis, this book and nutrition plan will be super simple for you. If you have some health and weight loss goals in mind, but you're not sure if keto is the right fit, put a check by the foods you can see yourself eating regularly. If you

KETOGENIC DIET

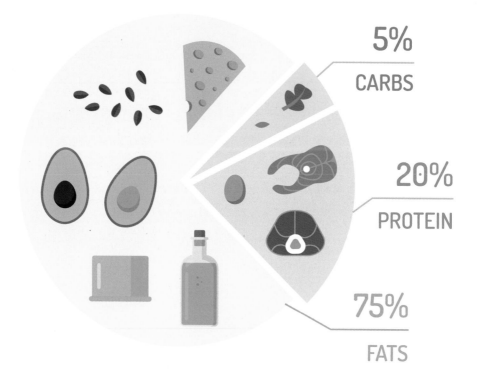

5%
CARBS

20%
PROTEIN

75%
FATS

choose at least ten of the foods under the "fats" heading, at least five foods under "carbo-hydrates," and at least four items labeled "protein," you will most likely have success on the keto nutrition plan. Keep in mind, this is a very general list and there are over 100 keto foods to choose from in chapter 2; however, this snapshot to the right is the basic foundation of the diet.

There are several ways to do keto and not all books exhibit the super simple way. We wrote this book to help you understand the ketogenic protocol and instruct you on how to get the fastest results possible with ease. In fact, you probably picked up this book because you have heard about the widely popular keto diet and how it has helped millions of people lose weight and improve overall health, yet you still feel like keto is probably

Fats	Carbohydrates	Protein
○ Avocado	○ Bell pepper	○ Boneless pork
○ Avocado oil	○ Blackberries	○ Lean cuts of beef
○ Bone-in pork	○ Blueberries	○ Lean fish (cod, sole,
○ Cheese	○ Eggplant	flounder, halibut, haddock,
○ Chicken or turkey (skin	○ Green vegetables	mahi mahi)
on)	○ Lettuces/leafy greens	○ Lean shellfish (shrimp,
○ Coconut oil	○ Raspberries	crab, clams, scallops,
○ Eggs	○ Squash	lobster)
○ Ground beef	○ Strawberries	○ Skinless chicken
○ Ham	○ Tomato	○ Skinless turkey
○ Herring		
○ Lamb		
○ Mackerel		
○ Nut butters		
○ Nuts		
○ Olive oil		
○ Olives		
○ Oysters		
○ Salmon		
○ Sardines		
○ Steak		

complicated. That is not the case! Keto can be super simple and the best part is the documented, short-term benefits of the ketogenic diet include a variety of positive health outcomes in addition to weight loss, including reduced blood sugar, triglycerides, and LDL (bad) cholesterol and increased HDL (good) cholesterol. Some studies have also suggested that the diet may have anti-aging, anti-inflammatory, and cancer-fighting benefits.

Super Simple Keto will help you achieve your weight loss and wellness goals safely and efficiently through a user-friendly ketogenic nutrition plan. In addition to offering a selection of six-ingredient (or less) unique keto recipes for variation and experimentation, the majority of this book coaches the reader on exactly what to eat to produce results as quickly and easily as possible. Even more important than fewer pounds on the scale, our intention for you is to improve your overall health and wellness via improvements in blood sugar, cholesterol, and triglycerides. Because of this, you will find that we focus our plan on the healthiest anti-inflammatory fats and advise against regular consumption of some common keto-approved foods such as bacon, hot dogs, and pork rinds.

Our super simple plan is so easy, and will reset your nutrition plan and rid you from your cravings for a high-sugar diet. You may achieve your desired initial results in the first thirty days, or you may continue this structured plan for up to six months. While there are no long-term studies beyond six months regarding the safety of keto, there are thousands of anecdotal scenarios which extend far beyond six months and suffer no ill effects.

There is a lot of fluff in many diet and nutrition books and we don't want to waste your time. You will fully understand how keto works and how to implement it into your own life by only reading chapters one through four of this book. Will you still want to read the rest? Yes! The additional chapters provide so much more variety and of course, all of the six-ingredient recipes, but if you're in a pinch and you need to get to know keto *now,* dedicate the next hour or two to **pages 1 to 28** and you'll be on your way. Congratulations—your new life is about to begin!

Chapter 1

Keto Boot Camp Part I: Simple Ketogenic Nutrition

Welcome to Keto Boot Camp! You may have picked up this *super simple* book because the ketogenic diet yields fast results for millions of people, but if you don't know much about the topic, it may seem daunting to learn. You will be instructed on everything you need to know about the keto lifestyle in these first two chapters. To fully understand the keto protocol, you need to know a little bit about nutrition and dietetics so that's what this boot camp chapter focuses on, but not to worry—it's going to be super simple. After you get the nutrition basics, the following chapter will focus on food, telling you everything you can (and can't) eat in easy-to-refer to charts.

The basic premise of the ketogenic diet is to get the body into the metabolic state of ketosis which causes your body to burn fat (instead of carbohydrates) for fuel. To accomplish this, you will need to eat a diet high in fat (but focus on healthy fats!), moderately low in protein, and very low in carbohydrates. To turn your gut into a fat-burning machine, there are guidelines to follow, however one should have a basic understanding of ketogenic nutrition to be successful.

Keto-Approved Foods

The keto protocol calls for high fat, moderate protein, and low carbohydrates so the foods you eat will need to reflect this nutrition profile. The following chapter will detail all of the foods you can and cannot eat when following the ketogenic nutrition plan. Generally speaking, you can eat green vegetables, some non-green vegetables, some extremely low-sugar fruits, nuts, seeds, eggs, some dairy, and oils. You cannot eat bread (or anything else with grains), pasta, beans/legumes, sugar, rice, corn, milk, or other items that are high or moderate in sugar or carbohydrates.

KETODIET FOOD PYRAMID

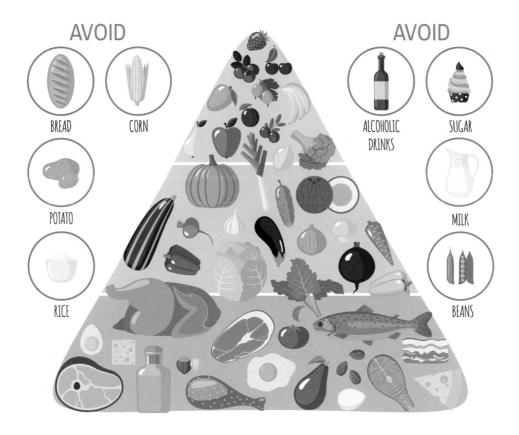

AVOID

BREAD

CORN

POTATO

RICE

AVOID

ALCOHOLIC DRINKS

SUGAR

MILK

BEANS

Macronutrients

You will hear this term (or "macros") a lot and the proper combination of them is the foundation of the keto diet, so it's important to have a clear understanding of macronutrients. Simply put, macronutrients are fats, proteins, and carbohydrates. They are required in larger amounts in the diet, hence the term "macro." Macronutrients are measured in grams such as 45 grams of fat, 30 grams of protein, or 15 grams of carbohydrates. Macronutrients are not to be confused with micronutrients, as micronutrients consist of vitamins and minerals and are needed in the diet in much smaller quantities, so they are measured in the smaller units of milligrams or micrograms.

Ketogenic Macronutrient Percentages

The keto diet calls for very particular percentages of macronutrients (fats, proteins, carbohydrates) to get the body into the metabolic state of ketosis which will help to turn your gut into a fat-burning machine. The keto macronutrient percentages range from 70 to 80 percent fat, 20 to 25 percent protein, and 5 to 10 percent carbohydrates. This means that most of your calories will come from fat, some will come from protein, and few will come from carbohydrates.

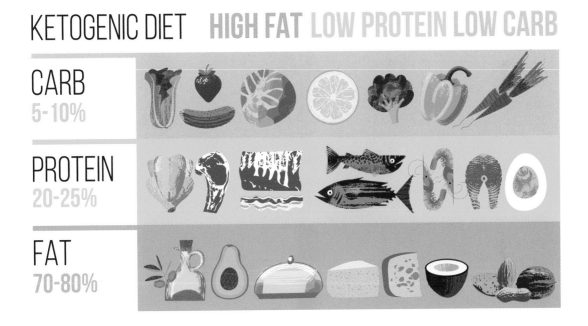

KETOGENIC DIET HIGH FAT LOW PROTEIN LOW CARB

CARB
5-10%

PROTEIN
20-25%

FAT
70-80%

Calories

As with any nutrition plan, calories in versus calories out will have a bearing on your weight loss and wellness success. It is important to know how many calories you require to hit your personal goals. There are several free online calculators which will reveal how many calories you should consume to get to your goal weight. Once you have determined how many calories you should be consuming, you can refer to the chart below to see how the keto macronutrients align with your caloric intake.

Total Calories	Fat Calories	Grams of Fat	Protein Calories	Grams of Protein	Carbohydrate Calories	Grams of Carbohydrates	Daily Total
1200 calories	840–960	93–107	120–240	30–60	60–120	15–30	1200 Calories 93–107 grams fat 30–60 grams protein 15–30 grams carbs
1500 calories	1050–1200	117–133	150–300	38–75	75–150	19–38	1500 Calories 116–133 grams fat 38–75 grams protein 19–38 grams carbs
2000 calories	1400–1600	156–178	200–400	50–100	100–200	25–50	2000 Calories 156–178 grams fat 50–100 grams protein 25–50 grams carbs
2500 calories	1750–2000	194–222	250–500	63–125	125–250	31–63	2500 Calories 194–222 grams fat 63–125 grams protein 31–63 grams carbs
3000 calories	2100–2400	233–267	300–600	75–150	150–300	38–75	3000 Calories 233–267 grams fat 75–100 grams protein 38–75 grams carbs

Net Carbohydrates Versus Total Carbohydrates

You will hear of "net carbohydrates" in the ketogenic world. Total carbohydrate limits found in the table above account for straight up carbohydrate totals as listed on the nutrition label. Net carbohydrates are found by subtracting the grams of fiber (which are indigestible carbohydrates) from the grams of carbohydrates. For example, a serving of cauliflower contains five grams of carbohydrates and two grams of fiber so you simply subtract two from five and that gives you three grams of net carbohydrates. Some circles in the keto community also advise to subtract grams of sugar alcohols (in addition to the grams of fiber) to get net carbohydrates. Other circles advise against this as many studies show that sugar alcohols actually do get absorbed into the blood stream to some extent, affecting blood glucose levels. One of our goals is to help kick the sugar habit so none of our recipes incorporate sugar alcohols, and you can simply subtract grams of fiber from grams of carbohydrates to get your net carbohydrate count. If you count total carbohydrates as per the nutrition label, you can follow the table above. If you choose to take the "net carbohydrate" route, an average rule of thumb to follow is to not exceed twenty-five grams of net carbohydrates per day.

Fats

When it comes to keto, people talk about carbohydrates a lot because one needs to keep them at a strict limit to get and remain in ketosis. Fats are just as important as all fats are not created equally. You will probably hear of the term "dirty keto" and that refers to the acceptance of having a fat free-for-all including unlimited unhealthy selections such as bacon, hot dogs, deli meats, pork rinds, and low-carbohydrate fast food. While you can have those items here and there if you choose, we do not recommend regular consumption of those products. Besides the fact that these above-mentioned items can be high in sodium, additives, and preservatives, they are also filled with fats that may contribute to bad cholesterol and cardiovascular issues.

To break it down in a super simple way, Omega-6 fatty acids are the most consumed in the western diet as they are found in processed foods by way of soybean oil, corn oil, and safflower oil, as well as cured meats. Because Omega-6 fatty acids are found in overly-consumed packaged foods, we get too many of them—far more than what our bodies require! We are in desperate need of a higher proportion of Omega-3 fatty acids, but those are harder to find since they are in fewer foods. Doctors and dietitians recommend having an Omega-6 to Omega-3 ratio of no more than 4:1 however, the average ratio in the United States is 50:1 which is a substantial unbalance. When the Omega-6 intake far outweighs Omega-3, inflammation and inflammatory disease can occur.[1] Adequate Omega-3 fatty acid intake is also critical as they are the only fatty acids which contain eicosapentaenoic acid (EPA) and docosahexaenoic acid (DHA). Together, EPA and DHA help to decrease inflammation and heart disease, while on its own, DHA is critical for brain function and eye health. Seafood, by leaps and bounds,

---

1   Calder, P. C. "Marine Omega-3 Fatty Acids and Inflammatory Processes: Effects, Mechanisms and Clinical Relevance," April 2015, https://pubmed.ncbi.nlm.nih.gov/25149823/.

is the best dietary source of DHA and is really the only food which will give adequate amounts of the fatty acid.

Unlike polyunsaturated Omega-3 and Omega-6, monounsaturated Omega-9 fatty acids are actually produced in the body so they are not technically needed in the diet. Research shows that several health benefits are associated with replacing inflammatory Omega-6 fatty acids with Omega-9s. One large-scale study found that higher Omega-9 intake reduced plasma triglycerides (fat in the blood) by nineteen percent and LDL ("bad") cholesterol by twenty-two percent in participants with type 2 diabetes.[2] Another study found that people who consumed high-monounsaturated fat diets had better insulin sensitivity, and less inflammation than others who consumed diets high in saturated fat.[3]

Needless to say, even though the ketogenic diet calls for high-fat, that statement is sometimes used in too much of a general manner. Fats are certainly not equal and should not be treated as such. For the healthiest and most effective outcomes, consciously opt for more Omega-3 and Omega-9 fatty acids since they are harder to find in the diet and the Omega-6 fatty acids will fall into place since those are the most common fats in a wide variety of keto foods. For your convenience, you can refer to the following chart to see where you can find the different fatty acids.

Foods with Omega-3 Fatty Acids	Foods with Omega-9 Fatty Acids	Foods with Omega-6 Fatty Acids
Anchovies	Almonds and almond oil	Corn oil
Chia seeds	Avocados and avocado oil	Cottonseed oil
Flaxseeds	Cashews and cashew oil	Soybean oil
Mackerel	Olives and olive oil	Standard mayonnaise
Salmon	Walnuts and walnut oil	Vegetable oil
Sardines		
Walnuts		

2   Garg, A; "High-Monounsaturated-Fat Diets for Patients with Diabetes Mellitus: a Meta-Analysis," March 1998, https://pubmed. ncbi.nlm.nih.gov/9497173/.

3   Finucane, O. M. et al.; "Monounsaturated Fatty Acid-Enriched High-Fat Diets Impede Adipose NLRP3 Inflammasome-Mediated IL-1β Secretion and Insulin Resistance despite Obesity," June 2015, https://pubmed.ncbi.nlm.nih.gov/25626736/.

Proteins

As with fats, it is best to choose the healthiest proteins. Also, some proteins have a substantial fat composition so it's beneficial to be aware of the healthiest proteins as those higher quality proteins will also have higher quality fats. For example, bacon, deli meat, and hot dogs are considered proteins but they also fall into the fat category, and those types of fats are best consumed in moderation. Higher quality proteins such as wild salmon and grass-fed organic beef will have far more omega-3 fatty acids, and less environmental toxins and additives than something such as deli meat.

Ketones in the Body

Some keto dieters want to track the state of progress by measuring the amounts of ketones the liver is producing to ensure the metabolic state of ketosis is being achieved. This is certainly not required but if you're curious how to do it, the following options are available. The three primary ways to measure ketones are via the blood, breath, and urine, and they are detailed below.

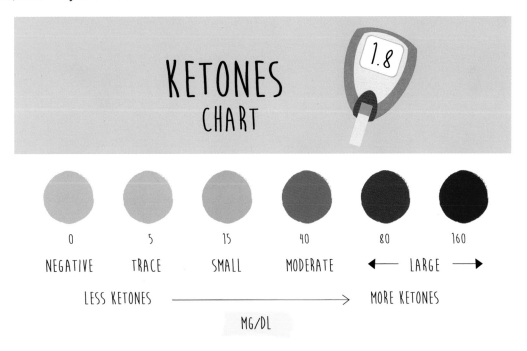

Blood Glucose Test: A simple blood test through the prick of a finger is the most accurate way to measure ketones. Be sure to wash your hands or disinfect with alcohol before the test, and it is helpful to prick the side of the finger where it's less sensitive. The ideal range to look for is between 0.5 and 5mM/L.

Breath Analyzer: Breath analyzers do not tell you your exact ketone level, however, they do provide a range to determine whether or not you are in ketosis. Some argue this form of testing is more reliable than the use of urine strips; however, it is not 100 percent accurate.

Urine Strips: Testing the urine measures the presence of acetoacetate (the first ketone produced in the body during ketosis). The darker the color of the test strip, the more ketones are present. This test can have false positives and negatives, so some in the keto community don't recommend this method as a preferred choice, however, many do employ it.

Grocery Shopping

It is common misconception that keto foods are hard to find, or one must shop at a specialty store. Keto-friendly foods can be found at most major grocery stores and many are even quite affordable! You will find an extensive list of all acceptable keto foods in the following chapter, however, generally speaking, keto nutrition consists of poultry, seafood, red meat, eggs, cheese, plain yogurt, nuts, nut butters, oil and butter, low-carbohydrate produce. Of course there may be some keto foods that are harder to find or more expensive but they certainly aren't required for success—see Chapter 19 to learn about niche keto foods you may not be aware of.

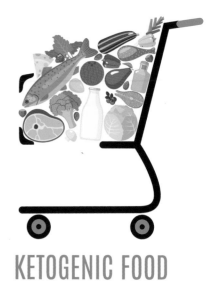

KETOGENIC FOOD

Sample One-Day Meal Plan

Let's put all of the information found in this chapter to use to create a realistic sample one-day meal plan. Following the menu, you will find a breakdown of calories, macronutrients, sodium, fiber, and sugar so you can see how everything falls into place.

Breakfast: Two whole eggs scrambled (using extra-virgin olive oil) and side of raspberries. Coffee with cream.

Snack: Macadamia nuts.

Lunch: Bun-less cheeseburger topped with avocado, lettuce, tomato, onion, and mustard.

Snack: Celery with almond butter.

Dinner: Salmon with coconut oil–sautéed spinach and broccoli.

Food	Calories	Fat	Protein	Net Carbs	Sodium	Fiber	Sugar
½ avocado	161	15 g	2 g	2 g	7 mg	7 g	0.5 g
70 percent lean ground beef (5 oz.)	465	40 g	20 g	0 g	95 mg	0 g	0 g
Eggs (2 whole)	156	10 g	12 g	1 g	124 mg	0 g	0 g
Almond butter (2 tbsp.)	196	18 g	7 g	3 g	2 mg	3 g	1 g
Broccoli (1 cup)	62	0 g	3 g	7 g	60 mg	5 g	1.5 g
Celery (2 stalks)	11	0 g	1 g	1 g	64 mg	1 g	0 g
Cheddar cheese (1 slice)	113	9 g	7 g	0 g	174 mg	0 g	0 g
Coconut oil (1 tbsp.)	117	14 g	0 g	0 g	0 mg	0 g	0 g
Cooked spinach (½ cup)	23	0 g	3 g	1.5 g	0 mg	2.5 g	0 g
Extra-virgin olive oil (1 tbsp.)	119	14 g	0 g	0 g	0 mg	0 g	0 g
Lettuce, tomato, onion, mustard garnish	25	0 g	1 g	3 g	120 mg	2 g	1 g
Macadamia nuts (¼ cup)	240	25 g	3 g	2 g	2 mg	3 g	0 g
Raspberries (½ cup)	33	0 g	0 g	3 g	0 mg	4 g	2.5 g
Salmon (6 oz.)	300	18 g	28 g	0 g	85 mg	0 g	0 g
Totals	**2,021 c**	**163 g**	**87 g**	**24 g**	**733 mg**	**28 g**	**7 g**

We hope Keto Boot Camp Part I has given you the basic understanding and foundation of the ketogenic protocol. Simply put, make sure you're consuming 70 to 80 percent fat (focus on those healthy fats!), 10 to 20 percent protein, and 5 to 10 percent carbohydrates. This regimen will put you on the fast track to ketosis and weight loss, but remember it's not required to measure your ketones. To see exactly what you can (and can't) eat, read on to Keto Boot Camp Part II.

Chapter 2

Keto Boot Camp Part II: Everything You Can (and Can't) Eat

This chapter is your go-to guide for everything you can and can't eat for keto. The meal plans found in coming chapters do not include every single item in the following "can" list, however, plenty of options are listed in case you are looking for a variety of additions. We urge you to eat the healthiest keto-approved foods as we would like you to achieve overall well-being in addition to your weight loss goals.

Vegetables

If you're unsure of which vegetables are best when making a grocery run, sticking to selections that are green is a rule to keep in mind. If you don't see your favorite(s) on the list, you can add them to the "can" category if green in color. If they are not green, check to see if each serving has five grams or less of net carbohydrates.

A Note About Organic Produce

It is always best to purchase as much organic produce as possible to avoid toxins and pesticides, but it can get pricey! There is a small handful of keto-approved vegetables and fruits that fall into the "dirty dozen" category, meaning they have the highest levels of pesticides. If possible, it is best to purchase the organic variations of these "dirty dozen" selections, and we have highlighted those for you.

A Note About Onions

A 100-gram (⅔ cup) serving of onions/shallots can have as much as 17 grams of carbohydrates, however, the manner in which one typically eats onions calls for much less than 100 grams. When sprinkling onions on a salad or sautéing shallots for a sauce, the carbohydrate count is still low enough to be keto-approved. If you're eating a roasted vegetable mixture and one component is onion, try not to exceed more than ½ cup of the onions.

Fruits

Some low-sugar fruits are allowed on the ketogenic plan, and some are so low in sugar that we may think of them as vegetables as opposed to fruits. Many fruits such as pineapple, mango, and grapes contain high amounts of fructose and fructose affects our bodies in a similar manner as table sugar, so it is imperative to eliminate high-glycemic fruits while adhering to the keto plan. Below are approved fruits for you to incorporate in your nutrition plan.

A Note About Berries

Berries are the higher-sugar and higher-carbohydrate selections of keto-approved fruits, however, they are packed with essential micronutrients, fiber, and antioxidants, so they are a healthy addition to anyone's diet. Since we are trying to remain extremely low in sugar and carbohydrates, this table will help you be mindful of your berry intake.

50-gram (½ cup) serving		
Berry Type	Total Carbs	Net Carbs
Blackberries	5 grams	2.5 grams
Raspberries	6 grams	2.5 grams
Strawberries	4 grams	3 grams
Blueberries	10.5 grams	8.5 grams

Vegetables	Fruits
○ Artichokes	○ Avocados
○ Arugula	○ Bell peppers (any color)
○ Asparagus	○ Blackberries
○ Bok choy	○ Blueberries
○ Broccoli	○ Cucumbers/pickles
○ Broccoli rabe	○ Eggplant
○ Brussels sprouts	○ Lemons
○ Cabbage/sauerkraut	○ Limes
○ Cauliflower	○ Olives
○ Celery	○ Pumpkin
○ Chard	○ Raspberries
○ Chicory greens	○ Spaghetti squash
○ Endive	○ Strawberries
○ Fennel bulb	○ Tomatoes
○ Green beans	○ Zucchini
○ Hot peppers	
○ Kale	
○ Kohlrabi	
○ Lettuces	
○ Mushrooms	
○ Onions	
○ Radishes	
○ Seaweed	
○ Spinach	
○ Swiss chard	
○ Watercress	

A Note About Eggs

Despite being a nutritious whole food, in 1968, the American Heart Association announced that all individuals should eat no more than three eggs per week due to their cholesterol content. Eggs also include invaluable vitamins and minerals, including vitamins B2, B5, B7, B12, and D, as well as omega-3 fats, high-quality protein, choline, iodine, selenium, and zinc. Because eggs contain cholesterol, they have been labeled as an unhealthy food that will contribute to raised LDL (bad) cholesterol and therefore, result in putting one at higher risk for heart disease. In 2015, the restriction of egg intake was eliminated from US dietary guidelines since there is lacking evidence that cholesterol from egg consumption actually causes heart disease. Many mainstream recommendations urge to consume cereal or oatmeal for breakfast due to being "heart healthy" despite the fact that those selections raise blood sugar (while eggs do not), but studies have shown that eating two eggs for breakfast in place of oatmeal reflects no change or increase in biomarkers related to heart disease.[1] In fact, more than fifty years of research has shown that the cholesterol in eggs has very little impact on LDL cholesterol levels, and is not associated with increased cardiovascular disease risk. Moreover, egg intake compensates for an array of common nutritional inadequacies, contributing to overall health and lifespan.[2]

---

1   Missimer, A., D. DiMarco, C. Andersen, A. Murillo, M. Vergara-Jiminez, and M. Fernandez. "Consuming Two Eggs per Day, as Compared to an Oatmeal Breakfast, Decreases Plasma Ghrelin While Maintaining the LDL/HDL Ratio." NCBI. February 01, 2017. Accessed April 27, 2019. https://www.ncbi.nlm.nih.gov/pmc/articles/PMC5331520/.

2   McNamara, Donald. "The Fifty Year Rehabilitation of the Egg." NCBI. October 2015. Accessed April 27, 2019. https://www.ncbi.nlm.nih.gov/pmc/articles/PMC4632449/.

Proteins

You will find a variety of keto-friendly animal proteins in this section and some selections can also double as fats as they are high in both protein and fat macronutrients. All animal proteins that have a substantial fat content are marked as such for your convenience.

Nuts, Seeds, Nut Butters, Seed Butters

Some nuts and seeds are lower in carbohydrates and higher in fat, making them better keto choices, however, all selections below are allowed on the keto nutrition plan. The lowest-carbohydrate selections are Brazil nuts, macadamia nuts, and pecans, while the highest in carbohydrates are cashews and pistachios. All others fall somewhere in between.

Poultry

- ○ Chicken
- ○ Chicken with skin
- ○ Duck
- ○ Game hen
- ○ Pheasant
- ○ Quail
- ○ Rabbit
- ○ Turkey
- ○ Turkey with skin

Eggs

- ○ Chicken eggs
- ○ Duck eggs
- ○ Goose eggs
- ○ Quail eggs

Red Meat

- ○ Beef
- ○ Boar
- ○ Buffalo
- ○ Elk
- ○ Goat
- ○ Lamb
- ○ Pork/Bacon/Sausage
- ○ Venison

Seafood

- ○ Anchovies
- ○ Bass
- ○ Carp
- ○ Catfish
- ○ Clams
- ○ Cod
- ○ Crab
- ○ Flounder
- ○ Haddock
- ○ Halibut
- ○ Herring
- ○ Lobster
- ○ Mackerel
- ○ Mussels
- ○ Octopus
- ○ Oysters
- ○ Prawns
- ○ Salmon
- ○ Sardines
- ○ Scallops
- ○ Snails
- ○ Snapper
- ○ Sole
- ○ Swordfish
- ○ Trout
- ○ Tuna
- ○ Walleye

Dairy

- ○ Butter and ghee (clarified butter)
- ○ Cheeses
  - *Blue cheese*
  - *Brie*
  - *Camembert*
  - *Cheddar*
  - *Cottage cheese (full-fat)*
  - *Cream cheese (full-fat)*
  - *Feta*
  - *Goat cheese*
  - *Gouda*
  - *Gruyère*
  - *Mascarpone*
  - *Mozzarella*
  - *Muenster*
  - *Parmesan*
  - *Provolone*
  - *Ricotta*
  - *Swiss*
- ○ Greek yogurt (full-fat)
- ○ Half-and-half
- ○ Heavy whipping cream
- ○ Kefir
- ○ Sour cream (full-fat)

Nuts and Seeds

- ○ Almonds
- ○ Brazil nuts
- ○ Cashews
- ○ Coconut (unsweetened)
- ○ Hazelnuts
- ○ Macadamia nuts
- ○ Peanuts
- ○ Pecans
- ○ Pili nuts
- ○ Pine nuts
- ○ Pistachios
- ○ Walnuts
- ○ Chia seeds
- ○ Flax seeds
- ○ Hemp seeds
- ○ Poppy seeds
- ○ Pumpkin seeds
- ○ Sesame seeds
- ○ Sunflower seeds
- ○ Almond butter
- ○ Cashew butter
- ○ Hemp seed butter
- ○ Macadamia butter
- ○ Peanut butter
- ○ Pecan butter
- ○ Sesame seed butter
- ○ Walnut butter

Cooking Oils and Fats			
Type	Smoke Point	Uses	Health Benefits
Avocado oil	520°F	Ideal for grilling, roasting, and pan-frying due to high smoke point. Can also be drizzled on salads and vegetables, or as a mayo replacement to add creaminess to dressings, sauces, and dips.	Monounsaturated fat to promote good cholesterol and heart health. Provides vitamin E, antioxidants, and healthy fats.
Coconut oil	350°F	Roasting at low temperatures, baking, smoothie, shake, or coffee addition. Can be substituted in for butter and other oils with a 1:1 ratio.	Provides easily absorbed medium chain fatty acids (MCTs) which are conducive for ketosis. Anti-inflammatory properties and beneficial for gut health.
Grass-fed butter	300 to 350°F	Used for low-heat cooking of eggs, fish, or shellfish. Topper for steak, roasted veggies, or keto chaffles.	Grass-fed butter has a higher composition of omega-3 fatty acids compared to grain-fed butter. Omega-3s are beneficial for heart and brain health, and cholesterol.
Grass-fed ghee	485°F	Used for sautéing meat, poultry, seafood, and vegetables. Can replace butter in most recipes, or be used as a spread.	Ghee is clarified butter so it is lactose- and casein-free, while still having a buttery taste and texture.
Medium Chain Triglyceride (MCT) oil	320°F	Used as a supplement and not typically for cooking. Ingredient in salad dressings, smoothies, shakes, and keto coffee.	Higher amount of MCTs than coconut oil—these saturated fats are easily digested and conducive for achieving ketosis. Beneficial for energy, and the feeling of satiety.
Olive oil	325-405°F	Low and medium heat cooking; "finishing oil" for flavor; salad dressings; marinades; drizzling over lettuces and vegetables.	High in monounsaturated fats which is linked to lower blood pressure and cholesterol. Consumption linked with improved cognitive health and blood vessel function, and the manufacturing process does not employ chemicals.
Walnut oil	320°F	Not ideal for cooking due to low smoke point. Can be added to shakes, smoothies, dressing, sauces, and keto coffee.	Good source of omega-3 fats which is beneficial for heart, eye, and brain health. The fats found in walnut oil can help to reduce bad cholesterol and increase good cholesterol.

Dressings and Sauces

There are many dressings and sauces that are allowed on the keto nutrition plan. The following premade selections can be found in most grocery stores but make sure to check the ingredients label to ensure they have no (or very little) sugar—ketchup and marinara tend to be problematic, but check the labels for any premade item. If you prefer to make your own dressings and sauces, please refer to Chapter 24.

Wine and Liquor

You can still participate in happy hour or have an adult beverage after a long day of work while on your keto plan. While some alcoholic drinks are packed with sugar and carbohydrates, others have the proper macros to fit into your nutrition plan if consumed in moderation. Having one (or sometimes two) of the following low-sugar and low-carbohydrate beverages, occasionally, won't sabotage your goals.

You may be pleasantly surprised that such a large variety of foods is allowed on the ketogenic nutrition plan. And of course, you are not required to use all of these foods, but they are available if you should choose to add them to your grocery cart.

Now, here are the foods to eliminate. The two common denominators which put foods on the exclusion list are sugar and carbohydrate contents that are too high for the ketogenic protocol. If you are unsure if you're allowed to use a food not found on this list, simply look at the carbohydrate content on the nutrition label. Given that on average you'll be staying under 50 grams of total carbohydrates per day, you will probably want to avoid any foods that have more than 8 grams of carbohydrates per serving. Of course this will depend on your total planned carbohydrate intake for the day—you may be able to get away with a serving of food that has more than 8 grams of carbohydrates if you plan your other portions accordingly.

Condiments

- Aioli
- Alfredo
- Béarnaise
- Blue cheese dressing
- Buffalo sauce
- Caesar dressing
- Gorgonzola sauce
- Hollandaise
- Hot sauce
- Italian dressing
- Ketchup
- Marinara sauce
- Mayonnaise
- Mustard
- Pesto
- Ranch dressing
- Soy sauce
- Sriracha
- Tzatziki

Miscellaneous Pantry Items

- Anchovy paste
- Apple cider vinegar
- Balsamic vinegar
- Bouillon cubes
- Broth
- Capers
- Chocolate (at least 75 percent cacao)
- Coconut cream
- Coconut milk (full-fat)
- Curry paste
- Fish sauce
- Red wine vinegar
- Tomato paste (low-carb, sugar-free)
- Vanilla extract

Red Wine

- Cabernet sauvignon
- Merlot
- Petite sirah
- Pinot noir
- Syrah
- Zinfandel

White Wine

- Albarino
- Brut champagne
- Chardonnay
- Pinot blanc
- Pinot grigio
- Sauvignon blanc

Liquor*

- Brandy
- Gin
- Rum
- Tequila
- Vodka
- Whisky

*The best keto mixers are club soda, plain sparkling water, and lime juice.

Foods to Eliminate

Bagels
Beans and lentils
Cake
Candy
Cereal
Commercial granola bars
Cookies
Corn
Cow's milk
Crackers
Croissants
Donuts
Fruit juice and other sugary beverages
Ice cream
Muffins
Pita bread
Pita chips
Pizza crust
Potato chips
Potatoes
Rice
Soda
Tortilla
White and whole wheat bread
White and whole wheat flour
White and whole wheat pasta

Chapter 3

How to Prepare Your
Super Simple Keto Kitchen

You may be surprised by the large variety of keto-approved foods provided in the previous chapter, and you may even be overwhelmed. While they are all options that can be used for the keto nutrition plan, you probably won't incorporate them all. While this can of course vary based on food preferences, this chapter serves as a general guide for how to prepare your keto kitchen.

There are some simple staple ingredients to have in your kitchen at all times and they are so basic they will not count towards the maximum six-ingredient total found in each recipe. These ingredients can be found in most grocery stores, have long shelf or refrigerator lives, and they are inexpensive—you likely have many or all of them already. You will be reminded of this list of required staples at the beginning of each recipe chapter.

Next you'll want to have a foundation of easy grab-and-go keto foods that can be thrown together for quick snacks or small meals. These foods also have relatively long shelf and refrigerator lives (at least three weeks) since we don't

Required Kitchen Staples (will not be counted in the six-ingredient recipes)

Your favorite oil(s)
Butter
Salt
Pepper
Garlic (dried powder or fresh cloves)
Water

Common Fresh Fare

Avocados
Beef
Bell peppers
Blueberries
Fresh fish and shellfish
Green vegetables
Leafy greens
Onions
Pork
Poultry
Raspberries
Strawberries
Tomatoes
Wild game

want to pack your kitchen with easily-spoiled fare. In addition, you don't want to always have to depend on preparing meals since it can be inconvenient, and eating small snacks throughout the day can help fend off hunger. If you don't enjoy one or some of the following foods or you have a similar option you prefer, feel free to omit.

When it comes to fresher foods which need to be prepared, the most popular and effective keto options to have in the house are produce and proteins. These have much shorter refrigerator lives so it's important to buy limited amounts based on meals needed throughout the week. If the expiration date on the proteins is approaching, either freeze, or cook and refrigerate to preserve for another five days.

One of the most widespread negative claims about the keto diet is regular use of red meat and processed meats. Reason being that red and processed meats can cause inflammation. Inflammation occurs when the body raises its production of white blood cells, immune cells, and cytokines that help fight infection. Chronic, long-term inflammation can occur internally without any detectable symptoms. This type of inflammation can fuel afflictions such as diabetes, heart disease, fatty liver disease, and cancer. You can certainly adhere to the ketogenic

Suggested Keto Staples

Avocados
Bell peppers
Berries (strawberries, blueberries, raspberries, blackberries)
Brazil nuts
Broccoli
Canned chicken, salmon, and tuna
Cheese
Chili peppers
Coffee
Cottage cheese
Cream
Cream cheese
Dark chocolate (at least 75 percent)
Deli chicken and turkey
Eggs (hard-boil ahead of time for an on-the-go snack)
Fatty Fish (salmon, herring, mackerel, anchovies, sardines)
Green Tea
Macadamia nuts
Mayonnaise (avocado oil or regular)
Mushrooms
Mustard
Olive oil
Olives
Pecans
Pickles
Plain Greek yogurt
Salami
Sauerkraut
Sparkling water
Tea leaves/bags
Tomatoes
Turmeric
Vinegar

nutrition plan without those foods, but if you prefer to incorporate them in moderate fashion, we strongly suggest our keto staples provided also be part of your *Super Simple Keto* kitchen.

Despite the fact that the keto diet includes a few inflammatory foods, if implemented in a healthy manner, it can be far more anti-inflammatory than the standard American diet. Sugar, high-fructose corn syrup, refined carbohydrates such as bread, cereal, pasta, crackers, chips, vegetable oils, trans fats, and alcohol are some of the most inflammation-promoting culprits in the food supply. Ironically, even though the keto diet is known for being "meat-heavy," thus being inflammatory, you can moderately incorporate meats while counterbalancing with an array of keto-approved foods which actually combat inflammation. We strongly suggest stocking your *Super Simple Keto* kitchen with these healthy, anti-inflammatory staples which are beneficial to anyone's nutrition plan.

Suggested Keto Budget Staples

Bell peppers	Green vegetables
Butter	Ground beef/chicken/turkey
Canned salmon and tuna	Leafy greens
Chicken/turkey drumsticks	Mushrooms
Chicken/turkey thighs	Olive oil
Cottage cheese	Plain yogurt
Cream	Some brands of bacon and deli meats
Cucumbers	Some cheeses
Eggplant	Tomatoes
Eggs	Zucchini/squash
Fresh shrimp	

The Budget Keto Kitchen

Can keto be expensive? Yes! Does it have to be to make it work and to get some serious results? No way! Some pricey keto foods such as Macadamia nuts, grass-fed steak, or fresh raspberries could lead one to believe that all keto-approved foods are expensive. While some are expensive, the majority of all keto-approved foods are either moderately or low-priced. To the left is a list of the least expensive keto foods to stock your kitchen with, and this single grocery list consists of enough foods for a complete keto nutrition plan, so with these groceries alone, one could construct a successful (and cheap!) keto plan.

If you're thinking there isn't enough variety for a keto plan on a budget (who doesn't love a nice steak or a piece of salmon?), here's something to consider. Giving up the standard American diet means giving up a lot of expensive grocery items, so you will have money to allocate to keto foods when you're not buying so many expensive non-keto staples that are typical in most households. On the next page is an analysis of the average annual costs for foods consumed at home and each highlighted category consists of non-keto foods, so that money spent can be allocated to your *Super Simple Keto* kitchen.

When examining the entire picture of all keto foods, as well as the money saved from staying away from mainstream packaged, carbohydrate- and sugar-ridden foods, the grocery costs of the keto nutrition plan versus others are quite comparable, even if some of the higher-priced items are included. The best news is, you are not required to add any hardware to your super simple kitchen as long as you have the typical pots, pans, and casserole dishes. You may want some food storage containers and/or some compartmentalized lunch boxes, but other than that, the only piece of kitchenware we may recommend is a mini waffle maker, only if you want to experiment with the chaffle (a waffle made from keto-approved foods) found in Chapter 13.

Average US Household Budget (2.5 people) for Food at Home of $3,935[6]	
Household Budget: Food at Home	Average Annual Amount
Nonalcoholic beverages	$384
Fresh fruits	270
Other canned and prepared foods	255
Fresh vegetables	236
Beef	219
Poultry	170
Pork	170
Bakery products	165
Milk	132
Sugar and sweets	143
Condiments and seasonings	138
Processed vegetables	130
Frozen prepared foods	130
Other meats	119
Cheese	125
Fish and seafood	122
Fats and oils	117
Potato chips and other snacks	115
Processed fruits	115
Bread	106
Cereals, ready to eat and cooked	94
Other cereal products (including rice, pasta, flour, and cornmeal)	91
Ice cream and related products	59
Eggs	56
Misc. dairy products	54
Cookies	49
Canned and packaged soups	45
Nuts	45
Crackers	39
Butter	24
Subtotal for Food at Home	3,935
Savings:	**$1874/year or $156/month**

---

6. Price, Sterling. "Average Household Cost of Food," June 19, 2020. https://www.valuepenguin.com/how-much-we-spend-food.

Chapter 4

The Super Simple Way to Get Started

An easy start-up process is key to starting any nutrition plan, as the preparation to begin some food plans is so daunting that many put off beginning in the first place! Keep in mind, we have many meal plans, batch-cooking techniques and recipes, meal preparation tactics, and unique keto foods to choose from so days to come will be far more varied, with the option to whip up interesting keto recipes. People are most likely to start a new regimen if it's easy, and that means not dealing with unfamiliar or hard-to-find foods, long preparation times, or expensive kitchen gadgets. The Super Simple Meal Planning Kit on the next page is the easiest formula to implement for formatting your keto meals. We urge you to use this kit for at least a week to learn the ropes of keto meal planning. If you stick to it only for the first seven days, you will see results on the scale that fast! And if you decide to continue with this meal planning system indefinitely, that is perfectly fine.

For meal examples which employ this chart, you will also find five breakfast, five lunch, five dinner, and five snack options—they are all keto-approved so the guesswork is taken out for you, and you'll be on your way to turn your gut into a fat-burning machine! For the next few days, pick a breakfast, lunch, dinner, and one or two high-fat snacks from the lists provided, or create your own meals using the chart on the next page.

SUPER SIMPLE KETO MEAL PLANNING KIT				
Pick a protein	Pick a low-carb produce (or two)	Add two or three fats	Pick one serving of low-sugar fruit per day (optional)	Optional condiments for any meal
Chicken	Asparagus	Avocado and avocado oil	Blackberries	Fresh or dried herbs and spices
Dairy-based protein (cottage cheese, Greek yogurt, kefir)	Bell pepper	Avocado oil mayo	Blueberries	Freshly squeezed lemon/lime
Eggs	Broccoli	Bacon	Raspberries	Hot sauce
Fish	Broccoli rabe	Cheese	Strawberries	Mustard
Ground beef	Brussels sprouts	Coconut milk		Sugar-free seasonings
Ground turkey	Cabbage	Coconut oil		Vinegar
Lamb	Cauliflower	Cream		
Plant-based protein (low-carb, low-sugar)	Cucumber	Eggs		
Pork	Eggplant	Grass-fed butter		
Shellfish	Green beans	Grass-fed ghee		
Steak	Leafy greens/side salad	High-fat, low-carb, low-sugar sauce or dressing		
Turkey	Mushrooms	MCT oil		
Venison	Onion (no more than two tablespoons per serving)	Nuts/seeds and nut/seed butters		
	Spaghetti squash	Olives and olive oil		
	Spinach	Regular mayo		
	Swiss chard	Walnut oil		
	Tomato			
	Zucchini			

Breakfast Options

Choose One

2-3 eggs cooked in oil your way, topped with cheese (optional) and avocado (optional) with side of berries or sliced tomatoes.

2–3 egg omelet with sautéed onions, bell pepper, and mushrooms, topped with cheese (optional) and avocado (optional).

2–3 eggs your way with 1–2 pieces of bacon.

Plain Greek yogurt or nondairy yogurt topped with berries and nuts or seeds.

Cottage cheese with berries or tomatoes.

Breakfast box to-go: 1 hard-boiled egg, 1 string cheese, 2–3 ounces smoked salmon, sliced avocado, handful favorite berries.

Lunch Options

Choose One

Green salad topped with chicken or steak, shredded cheese, sliced avocado, olives, oil and vinegar or store-bought ranch or blue cheese dressing (no sugar added).

1–2 cans of tuna or chicken mixed with mayonnaise, mustard, diced celery, and diced red onion. Eat on its own or use celery sticks to dip.

Deli sandwich lettuce wrap: fill one or two large iceberg lettuce cups with your favorite deli meats and cheeses, and any or all of the following: mayonnaise, mustard, avocado, tomato, onion, pickle.

Turkey burger or hamburger with no bun, topped with any or all of the following toppings: cheese, mayonnaise, mustard, avocado, tomato, onion, pickle.

Protein and fat platter: chicken, steak, or fish prepared with any of the following: melted cheese, sliced avocado, sautéed green vegetables, sauerkraut, green salad with oil and vinegar.

Dinner Options

Choose One

Sliced chicken, onion, and bell pepper sautéed in oil and store-bought tomatillo sauce (green sauce). Top with shredded cheese, sour cream, mashed avocado, and cilantro.

Steak topped with butter, paired with sautéed or roasted asparagus, and small side salad topped with oil and vinegar.

Salmon (or other fish) pan-cooked in grass-fed butter or ghee, paired with steamed cauliflower mashed with Parmesan cheese.

Hamburger (no bun) topped with cheese, mayo, mustard, lettuce, tomato, onion, and avocado paired with green vegetable of choice.

Lamb chops or lamb steak topped with Tzatziki Dipping Sauce (page 249) paired with green vegetable of choice.

High-Fat Snacks

Choose One or Two Per Day

Serving of nuts or seeds

Piece of cheese

Beef jerky

Celery dipped in nut butter or cream cheese

Red bell pepper slices with cream cheese and "Everything but the Bagel" seasoning

Hardboiled egg

2-3 squares dark chocolate (at least 75% cacao)

Small Keto Coffee (page 177)

Serving of olives

Serving of berries

Sliced tomatoes drizzled with olive oil and seasonings

Half avocado with melted cheese and salsa

Jicama or endive leaves dipped in mashed avocado

Sliced cucumber dipped in ranch dressing

Celery dipped in blue cheese dressing

Salami slices with cream cheese and sliced pickles

Deli turkey or ham rolled up with a piece of cheese

Coconut cream or half-and-half with raspberries

You can repeat meals if you like—for example, if you already have some eggs in the fridge and that means less grocery shopping, have eggs for breakfast on each day. Or if you want to make the tuna/chicken salad ahead of time and have it both days, that is fine too. We want to make the adjustment to your new nutrition plan as easy and inexpensive as possible. If this type of simplistic meal planning works for you (as it does for many!), you can use this system for as long as you like as these foods make up a solid foundation of the keto diet. If you want something new and more varied, keep on reading to later chapters!

Portions and Serving Sizes

We do not want you to count calories and weigh foods religiously—essentially, if you stick to the plans in this book, your keto macros will fall into place. On the next page is a portion guide to help you gauge a sensible portion that is most effective for results. Of course, this is a simplified list of keto foods; if you would like to see everything you can eat, refer back to Chapter 2.

Beverages

As with food, we need to stick to zero-sugar and/or extremely low sugar beverages. Water is always your best bet, but unsweetened coffee and tea with cream, coconut milk, coconut cream, MCT oil, coconut oil, butter, or ghee is also keto-approved. In addition, unsweetened sparkling water and bone broth are allowed, as well as one or two glasses of low sugar wine (per day) such as Cabernet Sauvignon, Merlot, Pinot Noir, Chardonnay, Pinot Grigio, and Sauvignon Blanc with dinner. Rum, whiskey, tequila, vodka, and gin are all keto-friendly, however, they cannot be combined with sugary mixers.

You May Want to Weigh In!

If you don't have a scale, it is beneficial to purchase one so you can track your progress, and it doesn't need to be anything fancy or expensive—just a simple scale that measures your weight. If you have access to a gym scale and you use the gym somewhat regularly,

Food	Calories	Visual Cue
Vegetables		
1 cup green vegetables	25 calories	1 baseball
2 cups leafy greens (raw)	25 calories	2 baseballs
Low-Sugar Fruits		
½ cup berries	45 calories	1 tennis ball
½ cup sliced tomato	15 calories	1 tennis ball
½ cup sliced bell pepper	15 calories	1 tennis ball
Fats		
½ cup sliced avocado	115 calories	1 tennis ball
1 tablespoon oil	120 calories	3 dice
1 tablespoon butter	100 calories	3 dice
1 tablespoon ghee	135 calories	3 dice
1 tablespoon mayonnaise	103 calories	3 dice
6 ounces salmon	300 calories	2 decks of cards
1 ounce nuts	160-205 calories	2 golf balls
2 tablespoons nut/seed butter	95-175 calories	1 golf ball
1 cup full-fat yogurt	150 calories	1 baseball
1 cup full-fat cottage cheese	200 calories	1 baseball
1 ounce olives	60 calories	10 whole olives
Proteins		
6 ounces chicken/turkey	200-275 calories	2 decks of cards
6 ounces steak	320 calories	2 decks of cards
6 ounces fish	150-310 calories	2 decks of cards
6 ounces shellfish	130-170 calories	2 hands full
6 ounces ground beef	360 calories	2 decks of cards

that can work too. Weight fluctuates throughout the day due to water and food consumption, as well as the clothing we're wearing, so we recommend weighing in first thing in the morning before getting dressed for the day. Jot your weight down or put it in your phone. When you complete your second weigh-in, consistency is key so if on your first weigh-in, you stepped on the scale before eating anything and before getting dressed in the morning, do the same for all future weigh-ins for the most consistent information.

Before Pictures

Sometimes we get just as much (or even more) results from inches lost, as opposed to the number on the scale. In addition to weighing in, take three before pictures—one frontward facing, one side facing, and one from behind. At the beginning of each month, it's a good idea to take the same three pictures so you can visually see the progress you have made. If you want to share your success, post on #eattokeepfit on Instagram and Facebook so everyone can see your results!

Congratulations for embarking on a *Super Simple Keto* journey. Remember to weigh yourself the morning of your first official day of food as you will probably see results after the first seventy-two hours. Keep in mind, although this keto meal planning kit and basic guidelines found in this chapter are simple, it is the foundation for the ketogenic diet. If you choose to keep using this system for longer than a few days, feel free—it works! You will be given more meal plans, recipes, and interesting keto cooking tricks to whip up delicious and unique fare in coming chapters.

Chapter 5

Super Simple Seven-Day Meal Plan Photo Guide

This seven-day meal plan is not only easy to put together, but you can also find all of these ingredients in most mainstream grocery stores. There are no recipes or measurements as this meal plan requires you to put only simple foods together with minimal preparation and cooking technique. If you are unsure of how to prepare each meal or snack, refer to the photo as an easy reference. As a reminder of food serving sizes, you can refer back to **page 27.**

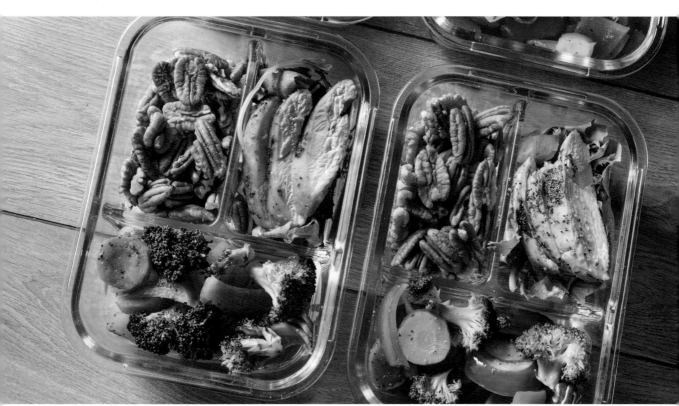

Day 1

Breakfast: Cottage cheese topped with berries and nuts

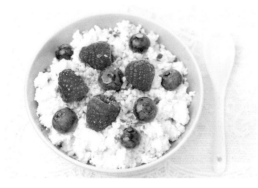

Snack: Celery with peanut butter

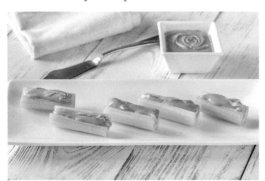

Lunch: Deli meat lettuce wrap

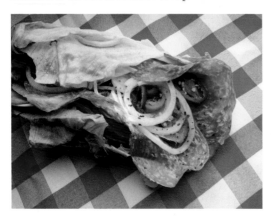

Snack: Serving of pork rinds

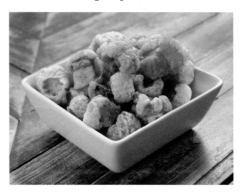

Dinner: Halibut with spinach and leeks

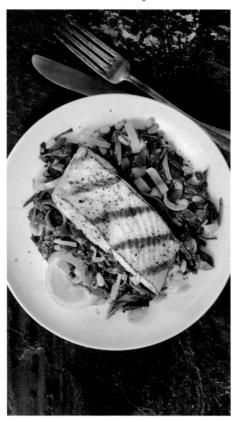

Day 2

Breakfast: Traditional bacon and eggs with sliced avocado

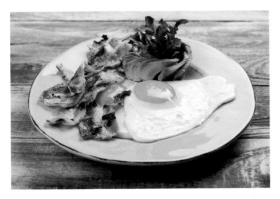

Lunch: Tuna salad

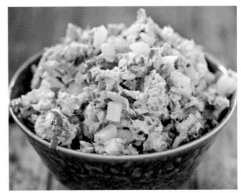

Snack: Serving of raspberries

Snack: Serving of nuts

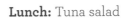

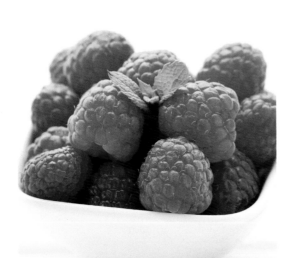

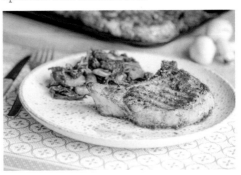

Dinner: Pork chop with sautéed spinach and mushrooms

Day 3

Breakfast: Cucumber slices with cream cheese and smoked salmon

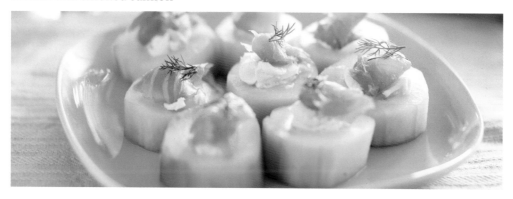

Snack: Hard-boiled egg

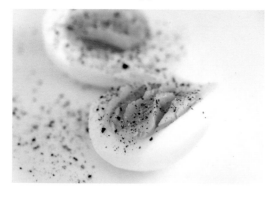

Snack: Piece of cheese

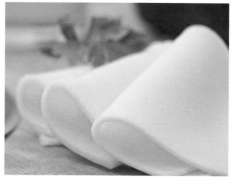

Lunch: Hamburger (no bun) with toppings

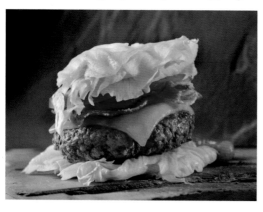

Dinner: Chicken with avocado salsa

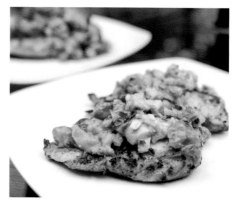

Day 4

Breakfast: Spinach and cheese omelet with tomatoes

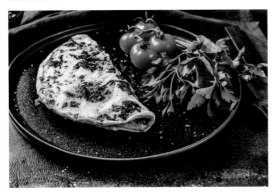

Snack: Serving of nuts

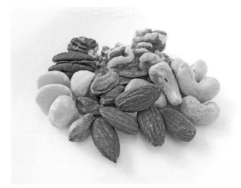

Snack: Serving of olives

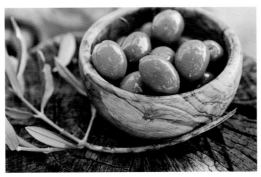

Dinner: Salmon with asparagus

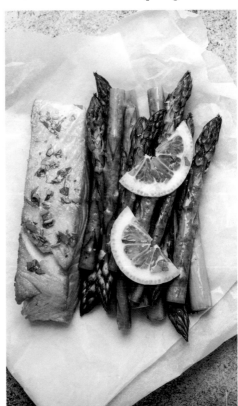

Lunch: Chicken wings with celery sticks and blue cheese dressing

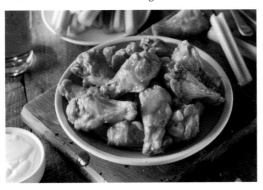

Day 5

Breakfast: Plain yogurt topped with strawberries and walnuts

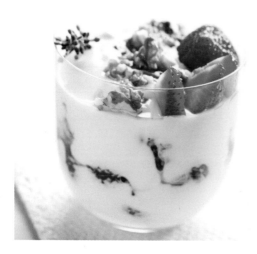

Snack: Keto coffee with coconut oil and butter

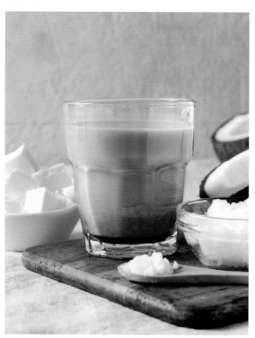

Lunch: Ground turkey in endive leaves topped with guacamole

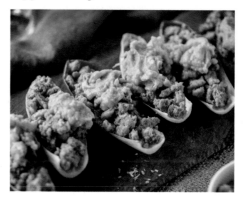

Snack: Deli meat wrapped string cheese

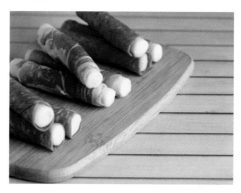

Dinner: Lamb chops with a side salad

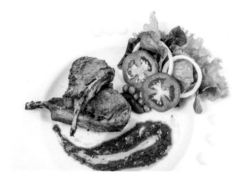

Day 6

Breakfast: Eggs, sausage, bacon, mushroom, and tomato platter

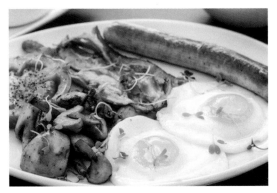

Snack: Bell pepper and cream cheese

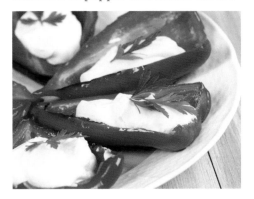

Snack: Serving of nuts

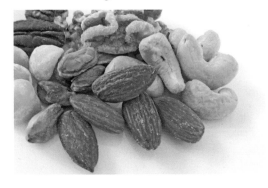

Dinner: Chicken and avocado salad

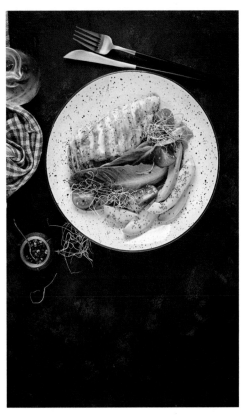

Lunch: Roasted turkey (skin on) with mashed cauliflower

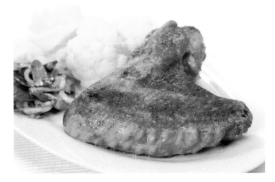

Day 7

Breakfast: Smoked salmon, egg, asparagus, nuts, and cheese Bento Box

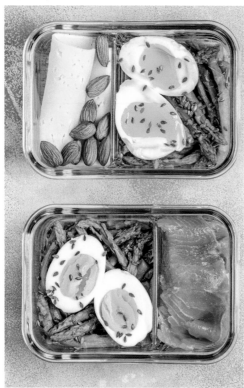

Lunch: Shrimp and avocado salad

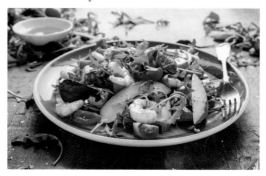

Snack: Serving of nuts

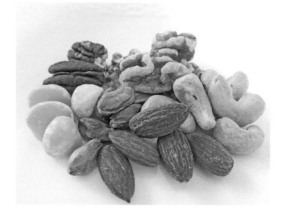

Snack: Cottage cheese topped with berries and nuts

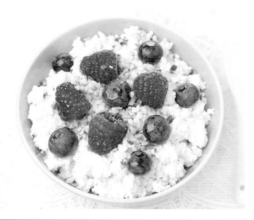

Dinner: Ribeye with green vegetables

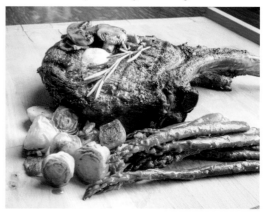

If you prefer some meals and snacks over others, choose your favorites and feel free to repeat them—including less variety will also cut down on grocery shopping time. Also, eating five times per day (three meals and two snacks) is not required. Only eat if you feel hungry, so if you're content with less meals and/or snacks, feel free to adjust this plan as needed.

Chapter 6

Keto Food Groups and Servings

If you're the type of nutrition planner who wants to know exact servings and amounts to eat, this chapter is for you. The types of calories you consume are just as (if not more) important as the amounts of calories you consume. Due to their macro- and micro-nutrient contents, the following food groups are essential for weight loss, steady blood sugar levels, and overall well-being, so we highly recommend making these guidelines an everyday goal to fulfill. It is important to note that you are *not* restricted to the foods listed on the next few pages; these food groups should take priority in your daily keto regimen, however, you will be able to incorporate other foods as well. For the complete list of acceptable *Super Simple Keto* foods, please refer back to chapter 2.

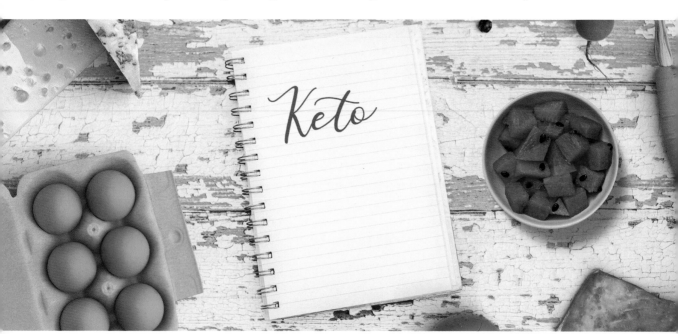

(1) Low-Glycemic Vegetables (2 to 3 servings)

Nutrient-dense vegetables are a good source of low-glycemic carbohydrates that will give you energy but help maintain even blood sugar levels. Several vitamins, such as vitamins A and C, and minerals such as iron and magnesium, are also found in these vegetables; plus many are high in calcium and fiber! If you don't see your favorite low-glycemic vegetable below, feel free to include it in your daily food regimen. The average amount of calories, carbohydrates, protein, fat, and fiber for the vegetables we provided are 12 calories, 2 grams of carbohydrates, 1 gram of protein, 0 grams of fat, and 2 grams of fiber in case you would like to compare your vegetable of choice to the ones in the recommended list.

Green Vegetable	Serving Size	Calories	Carbohydrates	Protein	Fat	Fiber
Arugula	½ cup	3	0 grams	0 grams	0 grams	0 grams
Bok choy	½ cup	5	1 gram	0.5 grams	0 grams	0 grams
Broccoli	½ cup	16	3 grams	1.5 grams	0 grams	1 gram
Brussels sprouts	½ cup	19	4 grams	1.5 grams	0 grams	1.5 grams
Cabbage	½ cup	9	2 grams	0.5 grams	0 grams	1 gram
Cauliflower	½ cup	13	2.5 grams	1 gram	0 grams	1 gram
Collard greens	½ cup	6	1 gram	0.5 grams	0 grams	0.5 grams
Kale	½ cup	17	3 grams	1.5 gram	0 grams	1 gram
Romaine lettuce	½ cup	8	0.5 grams	0.5 grams	0 grams	0 grams
Spinach (cooked)	½ cup	23	4 grams	3 grams	0 grams	2.5 grams

Whether you eat two or three servings per day will be based on your personal caloric needs. Since everyone is different, you can tailor your green vegetable needs based on your overall caloric intake requirements, as well as the keto macro-nutrient percentages you are targeting each day, given the amount of other consumed foods.

② Low-Sugar Nonfatty Fruits (0 to 2 servings)

Low-sugar fruits are another source of carbohydrates and energy. In addition, they provide even more micronutrients to add to the variety of benefits the low-glycemic vegetables boast. Try to incorporate tomato or red bell pepper in your servings of low-sugar fruits as they contain lycopene—a powerful antioxidant that is beneficial for heart health, sun protection, and reduced risk of certain cancers. Do not have more than one serving of berries per day in order to stick to your carbohydrate requirements. Please stick to the following low-glycemic fruit choices as the selections we have hand-picked for you are the lowest in sugar and remaining extremely low in sugar will be most advantageous for reaching your goals. The average amount of calories, carbohydrates, protein, fat, and fiber for the fruits we provided are 27 calories, 6.5 grams of carbohydrates, 1 gram of protein, 0 grams of fat, and 2 grams of fiber.

Low-Sugar Fruit	Serving Size	Calories	Carbohydrates	Protein	Fat	Fiber
Tomato	½ cup	16	3.5 grams	1 gram	0 grams	1 gram
Bell pepper	½ cup	15	3.5 grams	0 grams	0 grams	1 gram
Blueberries	½ cup	43	11 grams	0.5 grams	0 grams	2 grams
Raspberries	½ cup	33	8 grams	1 gram	0 grams	4 grams
Strawberries	½ cup	25	6 grams	0.5 grams	0 grams	1.5 grams
Blackberries	½ cup	31	7 grams	1 gram	0 grams	4 grams

Whether you eat one or two servings per day will be based on your personal caloric needs. Since everyone is different, you can tailor your low-sugar fruit needs based on your overall caloric intake requirements.

③ Summer and Winter Squash (0 to 1 serving)

Squash is mistakenly known as a vegetable or tuber but it's actually a fruit, and it is another source of carbohydrates that contain essential nutrients and antioxidants. Since the keto protocol requires us to remain extremely low in carbohydrates and sugar, it is important to note the lower carbohydrate variety of squash which is the summer squash: zucchini, zephyr, and cousa; however, zephyr and cousa can be hard to find in some grocery stores. Up to two servings per day are allowed for these varieties and up to one serving per day is allowed of the winter varieties (butternut squash, pumpkin, spaghetti squash, and acorn squash). Please stick to the choices below as other starches are too high in carbohydrates for the typical keto regimen. The average amount of calories, carbohydrates, protein, fat, and fiber for the starches we provided are 24 calories, 6 grams of carbohydrates, 1 gram of protein, 0 grams of fat, and 1 gram of fiber.

Squash Fruits	Serving Size	Calories	Carbohydrates	Protein	Fat	Fiber
Zucchini	1 cup	21	4 grams	1.5 grams	0.5 gram	1 gram
Zephyr	1 cup	19	4 grams	1.5 gram	0 grams	1 gram
Cousa	1 cup	20	4 grams	1.5 gram	0.5 gram	1 gram
Butternut squash	½ cup	32	8 grams	1 gram	0 grams	1.5 grams
Pumpkin	½ cup	15	4 grams	0.5 gram	0 grams	0 grams
Spaghetti squash	1 cup	31	7 grams	1 gram	1 gram	1.5 grams
Acorn squash	½ cup	28	8 grams	0.5 gram	0 grams	1 gram

Whether you eat zero or one serving per day will be based on your personal caloric needs, as well as the amount of other carbohydrates you have eaten or will plan to eat on the same day. Since everyone is different, you can tailor your squash needs based on your overall caloric intake requirements.

(4) Protein (3 to 5 servings)

Protein contains amino acids which are the essential building blocks of muscle and muscle burns fat, but not all proteins are created equal. It is imperative to consume high quality proteins (organic, grass-fed, and wild, if possible) that are unprocessed and have minimal preservatives, fillers, and environmental toxins. If you don't see your favorite protein below, feel free to include it in your daily food regimen. The average amount of calories, carbohydrates, protein, fat, and fiber for the proteins we provided are 116 calories, .5 grams of carbohydrates, 19 grams of protein, 4 grams of fat, and 0 grams of fiber.

Protein	Serving Size	Calories	Carbohydrates	Protein	Fat	Fiber
Eggs	1 whole egg (large)	78	0.5 grams	6 grams	5 grams	0 grams
Chicken (boneless/skinless)	3 ounces	90	0 grams	17 grams	1.5 grams	0 grams
Turkey (boneless/skinless)	3 ounces	120	0 grams	26 grams	1 gram	0 grams
Cod	3 ounces	70	0 grams	15 grams	1 gram	0 grams
Shrimp	3 ounces	90	1 gram	17 grams	1.5 grams	0 grams
Scallops	3 ounces	90	5 grams	17 grams	0.5 gram	0 grams
Wild salmon	3 ounces	143	0 grams	18 grams	8 grams	0 grams
Lean beef	3 ounces	158	0 grams	26 grams	5 grams	0 grams
Chicken with skin	3 ounces	190	0 grams	20 grams	11 grams	0 grams
Turkey with skin	3 ounces	129	0 grams	24 grams	3 grams	0 grams
Canned tuna (packed in water)	3 ounces	90	0 grams	20 grams	1 gram	0 grams
Boneless pork chops	3 ounces	115	0 grams	20 grams	4 grams	0 grams
Bone-in pork chops	3 ounces	150	0 grams	17 grams	7 grams	0 grams

Whether you eat three, four, or five servings per day will be based on your personal caloric needs. If you add your own protein to the list, be sure to avoid low-quality choices that have detrimental additives such as nitrates—items such as hot dogs, deli meats, and fast-food meats should be eliminated or severely limited.

⑤ Fats (8 to 12 servings)

This group contains the beneficial fats that include properties that assist with weight loss, increasing good cholesterol, reducing bad cholesterol, and maintaining even blood sugar levels. The average amount of calories, carbohydrates, protein, fat, and fiber for the healthy fats below are 116 calories, 1.5 grams of carbohydrates, 5 grams of protein, 11 grams of fat, and 1 gram of fiber.

Fatty Food	Serving Size	Calories	Carbohydrates	Protein	Fat	Fiber
Avocado	½ cup	117	6 grams	1.5 grams	11 grams	5 grams
Walnuts	14 halves	185	4 grams	4 grams	18 grams	2 grams
Wild salmon	3 ounces	143	0 grams	18 grams	8 grams	0 grams
Eggs	1 whole egg (large)	78	0.5 grams	6 grams	5 grams	0 grams
Extra-virgin olive oil	1 tablespoon	119	0 grams	0 grams	14 grams	0 grams
Coconut oil	1 tablespoon	121	0 grams	0 grams	14 grams	0 grams
Avocado oil	1 tablespoon	124	0 grams	0 grams	14	0 grams
Macadamia nuts	1 ounce	204	4 grams	2 grams	21 grams	2.5 grams
Brazil nuts	1 ounce	186	3.5 grams	4 grams	19 grams	2 grams
Fatty cuts of meat	3 ounces	158	0 grams	26 grams	15 grams	0 grams
Cream	1 tablespoon	29	0.5 gram	0.5 gram	3 grams	0 grams
Coconut milk	2 tablespoons	68	2 grams	1 gram	7 grams	1 gram
Olives	1 ounce	41	1 gram	0 grams	4 grams	1 gram
Cheddar cheese	1 ounce	113	0.5 gram	7 grams	9 grams	0 grams
Mozzarella cheese	1 ounce	78	1 gram	8 grams	5 grams	0 grams
Cottage cheese	½ cup	111	4 grams	12 grams	5 grams	0 grams
Grass-fed butter	1 tablespoon	100	0 grams	0 grams	11 grams	0 grams

Whether you eat eight, ten, or twelve servings per day will be based on your personal caloric needs, as well as the amounts of macronutrients consumed from other foods. Since everyone is different, you can tailor your healthy fat needs based on your overall caloric intake requirements.

If you're unsure of how to incorporate these foods into a meal plan, the keto select meal planning system found in chapter 18 will detail a variety of ways to meet the above recommended requirements. For the most simplistic way to achieve these servings, you can also refer back to chapter 4's *Super Simple Keto* Meal Planning Kit. If you want to get even more creative, the *Super Simple Keto* breakfast, lunch, and dinner recipes found in chapters 21 to 23 include a variety of these foods, incorporated into delicious meals.

Chapter 7

The Big Question: Is Keto Safe?

A s with any dietary lifestyle, there tend to be healthy and unhealthy ways to follow a particular nutrition protocol, and this certainly goes for keto, too. One of the primary guidelines of *Super Simple Keto* is to choose the healthiest fats possible. Fats found in foods such as avocado, extra-virgin olive oil, nuts, seeds, and wild salmon actually help promote good cholesterol. If one focuses on unhealthy fats such as inferior oils and processed meats, then it is possible that negative outcomes such as increased bad cholesterol and excessive sodium levels could occur. There are several studies which show that particular variations of the ketogenic nutrition plan (like the one exhibited in this book) are associated with improvements in good cholesterol, cardiovascular risk, and type 2 diabetes.[1]

Of course, there are still many unanswered questions about the keto diet. There are few studies on the long-term (more than six months) effects of following an extremely high-fat regimen. In addition, several variations of the keto diet exist, some much less healthy than others. For example, "dirty keto" is a term coined to characterize a free-for-all of any type of fats such as unlimited bacon, hot dogs, pork rinds, and bunless cheeseburgers, and that variation could certainly lead to unfavorable health outcomes.

Due to the complexities and unknowns of this fascinating nutrition plan, which dates back to 1923, we highly recommend that this protocol to be followed for a relatively short period of time (no longer than six months) to kickstart your weight loss goals and obtain freedom from the high-carbohydrate lifestyle. The documented, short-term benefits of the ketogenic diet include a variety of positive health outcomes in addition to

---

1   Kosinski, Christophe, and François R Jornayvaz. "Effects of Ketogenic Diets on Cardiovascular Risk Factors: Evidence from Animal and Human Studies." Nutrients. MDPI, May 19, 2017. https://www.ncbi.nlm.nih.gov/pmc/articles/PMC5452247/.

weight loss, including reduced blood sugar, triglycerides, and LDL (bad) cholesterol and increased HDL (good) cholesterol. Animal studies have also suggested that the diet may have anti-aging, anti-inflammatory, and cancer-fighting benefits. And while there are no long-term studies documenting the safety of the ketogenic protocol, thousands of anecdotal stories of dieters adhering to the keto diet for far more than six months have shown limited negative outcomes.

Weaning Off Keto

You may be wondering what to do after you have gotten closer to your weight loss goals, and you'd like to gradually go from keto to a more moderate nutrition plan. The wean-off strategy is called Almost Keto and it employs all the foods you have been working with in this book, however, the macronutrient composition will be different. Many say it's easier, healthier, and more sustainable for the long-term. In fact, you'll be cutting your fat intake substantially and the best news (for some) is that you will have more room for low-glycemic carbohydrates by way of green vegetables and low-sugar fruits. Essentially, you'll still eat the same keto-approved foods, however, your macronutrient percentages will change to be lower in fat and higher in carbohydrates. Your food plan will still be moderately low in carbohydrates and sugar, compared to the standard American diet, so you will still see your results progress and be maintained. Here is your "almost keto" macro chart (above), but if you'd like more extensive information on this nutrition plan, you can find it all in our book titled *Almost Keto*.

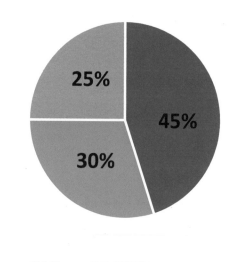

Almost Keto Macronutrients

25%

45%

30%

■ FAT   ■ PROTEIN   ■ CARBS

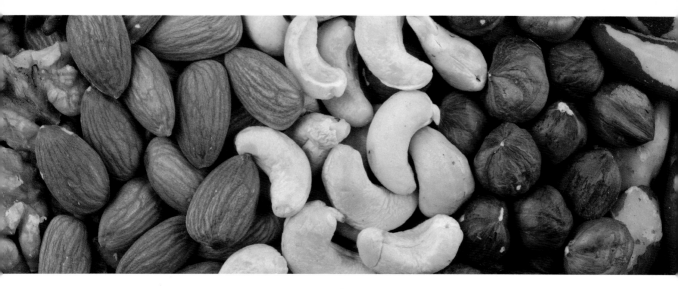

Keto Nutrients

One of the largest complaints about the keto diet is that it is devoid of essential nutrients—but this is false. Avoiding high-glycemic and high-starch carbohydrates such as bread, pasta, cereal, rice, and potatoes does not have to mean missing out on vitamins, minerals, and fiber as there is an array of those nutrients in other foods, despite the popular misconception that you need fortified processed foods to meet your micronutrient intake. For your convenience, you will find a variety of charts and tables below. They can be used as a handy reference where you can quickly find the nutrients you're looking for, a general guideline of how much of each nutrient you should consume on a daily basis, as well as the corresponding foods that boast each nutrient.

Mainstream dietary recommendations are strongly influenced by lobbying, funding, and food manufacturers, so when these types of vitamin and mineral charts are found on our governmental websites, the food source recommendations are comprised heavily of big-name processed foods that have fortified synthetic nutrients. Many of those foods consist of high-glycemic selections such as fortified juices, cereals, and breads, as well as other unhealthy foods such margarine and vegetable oil. We must ponder these recommendations and question them being based on nutrition science and truth, as opposed to funding from special interest groups. The following super simple macro- and micronutrient charts contain unprocessed, whole foods that have naturally occurring vitamins and minerals.

Vitamins

Vitamin	Function	Food Source	Daily Amount
Biotin	Metabolizes protein, fat, carbohydrates for energy. Beneficial for skin, hair, and nail health.	Avocado, cauliflower, eggs, liver, pecans, pork, raspberries, salmon, sunflower seeds, walnuts	30 mcg
Folate	Metabolizes protein and assists with red blood cell formation. Prevents birth defects (pregnant women should consume 600–800 mcg per day).	Arugula, asparagus, avocado, beef liver, broccoli, brussels sprouts, eggs, flaxseeds, kale, lemon, lime, walnuts	400 mcg
Niacin	Aids with nervous system functioning and digestion. Helps convert food into energy.	Anchovies, avocado, chicken breast, ground beef, liver, mushrooms, peanut butter, pork, salmon, tuna, turkey	20 mg
Pantothenic Acid	Helps the functioning of the nervous system and formation of red blood cells. Metabolizes fat and aids in hormone production.	Avocados, broccoli, eggs, cauliflower, portobello mushrooms, poultry, salmon, sunflower seeds, yogurt	10 mg
Riboflavin	Assists with general growth and development, red blood cell formation, and energy conversion from foods.	Almonds, beef liver, eggs, lamb, mushrooms, oysters, poultry, spinach, tahini, wild salmon, yogurt	1.7 mg
Thiamin	Converts food to energy and assists with nervous system functioning.	Asparagus, brussels sprouts, beef liver, nutritional yeast, macadamia nuts, pork, sunflower seeds, seaweed	1.5 mg
Vitamin A	Beneficial for vision, immune function, and reproduction. Assists with growth and development, as well as red blood cell, skin, and bone formation.	Broccoli, beef liver, butter, collard greens, eggs, goat cheese, kale, red peppers, romaine lettuce, salmon, spinach, trout	5,000 IU
Vitamin B6	Assists with nervous system, immune function, and red blood cell formation. Helps metabolize protein, fat, and carbohydrates.	Avocado, chicken, eggs, nutritional yeast, pork, ricotta cheese, salmon, tuna, turkey, spinach	2 mg
Vitamin B12	Helps convert food into energy and assists with red blood cell formation and nervous system function.	Beef, clams, eggs, nutritional yeast, sardines, salmon, seaweed, trout, tuna, yogurt	6 mcg

Vitamin C	Assists with immune function and wound healing. Combats free radicals and helps with collagen and connective tissue formation.	Broccoli, brussels sprouts, bell peppers, berries, lemon, lime, tomatoes	60 mg
Vitamin D	Regulates blood pressure and balances calcium. Promotes hormone production, bone growth, immune and nervous system function.	Beef liver, egg yolks, herring oysters, salmon, sardines, shrimp, tuna, responsible sun exposure	1,000 - 4,000 IU
Vitamin E	Strong antioxidant to combat free radicals. Supports immune function and blood vessel formation.	Almonds, avocado, Brazil nuts, broccoli, hazelnuts, peanut butter, pine nuts, rainbow trout, red sweet pepper, salmon, spinach, sunflower seeds	30 IU
Vitamin K	Supports strong bones and blood clotting.	Avocado, blackberries, blueberries, broccoli, brussels sprouts, cabbage, cauliflower, collard greens, kale, mustard greens, spinach, swiss chard, turnip greens	80 mcg

Minerals

Mineral	Function	Food Source	Daily Amount
Calcium	Supports nervous system and promotes bone and teeth formation. Assists with blood clotting, muscle contraction, hormone secretion, as well as constriction and relaxation of blood vessels.	Almonds, broccoli, canned salmon, cheese, cottage cheese, fresh salmon, Greek yogurt, kale, sardines, sesame seeds, spinach, turnip greens	1,000 mg
Chloride	Converts food into energy, and aids digest and fluid balance. Promotes acid-base balance and nervous system function.	Celery, lettuce, olives, seaweed, sea salt, tomatoes	3,400 mg
Chromium	Promotes protein, fat, and carbohydrate metabolism, and supports insulin function.	Basil, beef, broccoli, garlic, green beans, romaine lettuce, turkey	120 mcg
Copper	Promotes bone, collagen, and connective tissue formation. Assists with iron metabolism, energy production, and nervous system function. Antioxidant that combats free radicals.	Almonds, dark chocolate, kale, liver, lobster, oysters, sesame seeds, shiitake mushrooms, spinach, spirulina, Swiss chard	2 mg
Iodine	Supports thyroid hormone production, reproduction, and metabolism. Promotes general growth and development.	Cod, cottage cheese, eggs, Greek yogurt, green beans, kale, seaweed, shrimp, strawberries, tuna, turkey	150 mcg
Iron	Promotes growth and development, immune function, and energy production. Assists with red blood cell production, wound healing, as well as the reproduction system.	Beef, broccoli, clams, collard greens, dark chocolate, liver, mussels, oysters, pine nuts, pistachio nuts, pumpkin seeds, spinach, swiss chard, turkey	18 mg
Magnesium	Assists with blood pressure and blood sugar regulation, as well as heart rhythm stabilization. Promotes immune function, bone formation, energy production, and hormone secretion. Strengthens nervous system function, muscle contraction, and protein formation.	Almonds, avocado, Brazil nuts, chia seeds, collard greens, dark chocolate, flax seeds, halibut, kale, mackerel, pumpkin seeds, salmon, spinach	400 mg

Manganese	Promotes cartilage and bone formation, as well as wound healing. Assists with cholesterol, carbohydrate, and protein metabolism.	Almonds, black tea, collard greens, green tea, kale, mussels, pecans, pine nuts, raspberries, spinach, strawberries	2 mg
Molybdenum	Promotes enzyme production.	Almonds, bell pepper, celery, cod cucumber, cheese, eggs, fennel, Greek yogurt, liver, tomatoes, romaine lettuce, sesame seeds, walnuts	75 mcg
Phosphorus	Promotes hormone activation, energy storage and production, and bone formation. Supports acid-base balance.	Brazil nuts, carp, cheese, chicken, clams, cottage cheese, liver, pine nuts, pistachio nuts, pollock, pork, pumpkin seeds, salmon, sardines, scallops, sunflower seeds, turkey, yogurt	1,000 mg
Potassium	Supports heart function, blood pressure regulation, fluid balance, and nervous system function. Promotes general growth and development, muscle contraction, protein formation, and carbohydrate metabolism.	Artichoke, avocado, broccoli, brussels sprouts, butternut squash, clams, haddock, pumpkin seeds, salmon, spinach, sunflower seeds, Swiss chard, tomatoes, yogurt	3,500 mg
Selenium	Supports thyroid and immune function, as well as reproduction. Antioxidant that fights off free radicals.	Beef, Brazil nuts, chicken, clams, cottage cheese, crab, eggs, halibut, mushrooms, oysters, pork, salmon, sardines, shrimp, spinach, sunflower seeds, turkey, yogurt	70 mcg
Zinc	Promotes growth and development, protein formation, immune function, and wound healing. Supports nervous system function and reproduction, as well as taste and smell.	Almonds, beef, cheese, crab, eggs, green beans, hemp seeds, kale, pork, pumpkin seeds, lamb, mussels, oysters, pine nuts, sesame seeds, shrimp	15 mg

Now for a different perspective, below you will find micronutrients categorized by food group and macronutrient categories. Just like the above vitamin and mineral sources, these following foods are also keto-approved. The meal plans and recipes found throughout this book use these foods as primary ingredients to give you the best nutrition while hitting your *Super Simple Keto* plan requirements.

Food	Macronutrients	Micronutrients
Low-Glycemic Vegetables (broccoli, asparagus, Brussels sprouts, onion, cauliflower, spinach, kale, artichoke, collard greens, arugula, butter lettuce, romaine, Swiss chard, cabbage, radish, zucchini)	Carbohydrate	Vitamins A, C, E, and K; chromium, folate, fiber, pantothenic acid, vitamins B1, B2, and B6; manganese, selenium, pantothenic acid, niacin, potassium, phosphorus, choline, copper, Omega-3 fatty acids, calcium, and iron.
Low-Sugar Fruits (blueberries, blackberries, raspberries, strawberries, tomato, bell pepper)	Carbohydrate	Vitamins A, C, E, and K, fiber, biotin, molybdenum, copper, potassium, riboflavin, thiamin, manganese, fiber, vitamins B2 and B6, folate, niacin, phosphorus, carotenoids.
Other Low-Sugar Fruits (avocado, olives)	Fat	Vitamins C, E, and K, fiber, copper, potassium, vitamin B6, folate, Omega-3 fatty acids
Nuts and Seeds (almonds, pistachios, pecans, macadamia, Brazil nuts, pine nuts, walnuts, hazelnuts, sesame seeds, pumpkin seeds, chia seeds, flaxseed)	Fat and Protein	Vitamin E, vitamins B2 and B6, magnesium, zinc, fiber, biotin, copper, phosphorus, calcium, Omega-3 fatty acids
Poultry (organic chicken, duck, turkey)	Protein	Vitamins B2, B3, B6, and B12; niacin, phosphorus, choline, iron, selenium, zinc, phosphorus, choline, and pantothenic acid.
Other Poultry (eggs)	Protein and Fat	Vitamins A, D, E, K; choline, vitamin B12, thiamin, riboflavin, folate, zinc, copper, and selenium
Fish (wild salmon, halibut, sole, rockfish, trout, tuna, anchovies, mahi mahi, opah, sardines)	Protein and Fat	Vitamin D, vitamins B5, B6, and B12, magnesium, potassium, niacin, phosphorus, and selenium; omega-3 fatty acids
Shellfish (oysters, clams, shrimp, mussels, crab, lobster)	Protein and Fat	Vitamin B12, iron, zinc, copper, Omega-3 fatty acids
Meat (organic grass-fed beef, organic grass-fed lamb, venison, bison)	Protein and Fat	Vitamins B3, B6, and B12; Omega-3 fatty acids, selenium, iron, zinc, phosphorus, choline, and pantothenic acid.
Dairy (Greek yogurt, cheese, cottage cheese)	Protein and Fat	Probiotics, calcium, potassium, vitamin A, vitamins B2, B6 and B12, zinc, phosphorus, selenium, and magnesium.

As you can see, staple foods found in the *Super Simple Keto* plan offer an abundance of essential vitamins and minerals, despite the fact that many dietary recommendations suggest processed foods due to their synthetic nutrient composition. Some processed foods do, in fact, offer fortified vitamins and minerals; however, one can find several whole foods that offer naturally occurring nutrients with superior absorption rates. An added benefit is that when consuming the above-mentioned whole foods as opposed to fortified breads, cereals, pastas, and fruit juices, you will avoid high-glycemic carbohydrates that contribute to raised blood sugar levels and potential weight gain.

Chapter 8

The Super Simple Way to Ease into Keto (If You're Feeling Nervous)

While many keto followers strictly adhere to the proper macronutrient requirements to get and remain in ketosis, if you're nervous about making such a commitment, you're not alone. Loosely following some keto principles will certainly yield results—in fact, some keto dieters never actually get into the metabolic state of ketosis, but still reap the same rewards. The ketogenic diet is extremely low in sugar and carbohydrates and that is key since sugar and carbohydrates turn to fat, if not burned. Even if you're not adhering to the exact 5 to 10 percent carbohydrate requirement, if you can manage 15 to 25 percent, you will still be consuming less than half the carbohydrates found in the standard American diet and that in itself will create change. The following four strategies, which are characterized by the keto diet but can still be loosely followed (without the need for ketosis), will contribute to substantial health and weight loss efforts.

Consuming Less Sugar

Sugar consumption is the primary culprit of weight gain, type 2 diabetes, and a host of other ailments. The average American consumes 71 grams (or 17 teaspoons) of added sugar per day, which translates into 57 pounds of added sugar per year, per person. When one shifts from the standard high-sugar American diet to one that is very low in sugar, weight loss and blood sugar improvements will naturally follow.

Consuming Fewer Carbohydrates

Like with sugar, when one adopts a dietary regimen that is substantially lower in carbohydrates, results will follow. The average person consumes 260 grams of carbohydrates per day, so when that number is cut exponentially, less sugar will be consumed as carbohydrates convert into sugar, and sugar turns into fat if not burned.

Consuming Fewer Calories

Consuming less sugar and carbohydrates will, of course, lead to lower calorie consumption. When we eliminate or limit "filler" foods such as sugary beverages with a meal, dessert following dinner, and empty-calorie main courses and side dishes, we will naturally consume fewer calories, and these calories will be more nutrient-dense, providing the fuel we need for a healthy lifestyle.

Foods to Eliminate

Bagels
Beans and lentils
Cake
Candy
Cereal
Commercial granola bars
Cookies
Corn
Cow's milk
Crackers
Croissants
Donuts
Fruit juice and other sugary beverages
Ice cream
Muffins
Pita bread
Pita chips
Pizza crust
Potato chips
Potatoes
Rice
Soda
Tortilla
White and whole wheat bread
White and whole wheat flour
White and whole wheat pasta

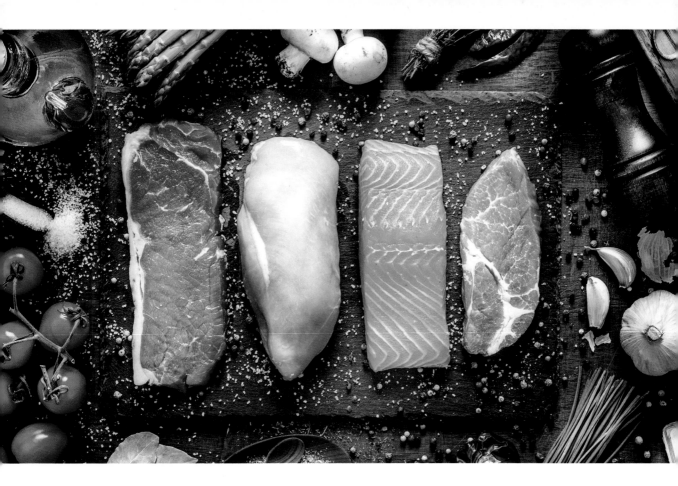

Eating Consciously

When a new dietary regimen is employed, we consciously choose to eat foods that are beneficial for weight loss and overall well-being, instead of maintaining the status quo of the standard American diet and eating what we always ate previously.

The most super simple way to ease into keto and follow the four above-mentioned strategies is to cut foods out of your nutrition plan that are not keto-approved. Referring back to chapter 2, we listed these foods that must be eliminated.

If you want to loosely follow keto, it's as simple as eliminating the above foods—you don't need to track your fat, protein, or carbohydrate intake whatsoever! Eating only keto-approved foods will result in an effective "almost keto" diet (described in the previous chapter) and you will still see drastic results. If you do choose the "almost keto" approach, you can focus on the following **Perfect 10** food groups.

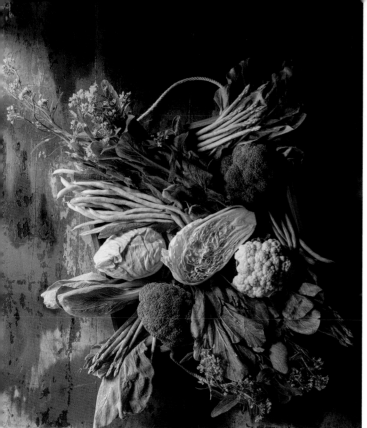

Green Vegetables

Nutrient-dense green vegetables should make up the majority of your carbohydrate intake and you can still eat several servings per day while remaining in the general lower-carbohydrate parameter. Nutrient-dense vegetables are low-sugar, unprocessed carbohydrate sources, and packed with micronutrients such as thiamine, riboflavin, folate, iron, magnesium, phosphorus, vitamin A, vitamin C, vitamin K, vitamin B6, vitamin C, calcium, potassium, and manganese; they are also chock-full of fiber which will aid in digestion and regular bowel movements.

Avocado

Avocados have special properties as they are one of the only fatty fruits! Like nutrient-dense vegetables, avocados provide a variety of essential vitamins and minerals, as well as fiber. According to the American Heart Association, the monounsaturated fat found in avocados can help reduce bad cholesterol levels, and the risk of heart attack and stroke. An added benefit is that when one consumes fat, the brain gets a signal to switch off the appetite. Eating fat slows the breakdown of carbohydrates, which helps keep sugar levels in the blood stable.

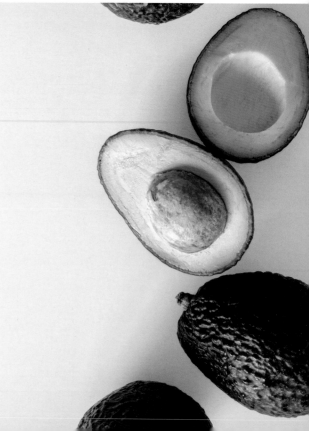

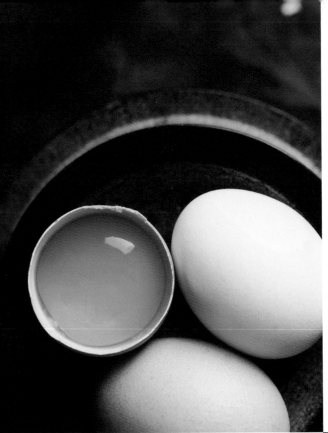

Eggs

Eggs are a nice mix of quality protein and omega-3 fatty acids. Some nutrition and medical circles advise to eat the egg white only but we urge you to keep that yolk. It is popular belief that the yolk doesn't have any protein; however, it does contain 2.7 grams which is 45 percent of the entire egg's protein composition. The yolk also boasts the superior omega-3 fatty acids, vitamins A, D, E, B12, and K, riboflavin, folate, and iron. Although eggs have been demonized in the past for containing cholesterol, numerous recent studies have cited a general consensus that cholesterol, primarily from egg yolks, poses very little risk for adverse effects on LDL (bad) cholesterol levels.[1]

1   Griffin, BA. "Eggs: Good or Bad?" NCBI. August 1, 2016. Accessed April 6, 2019. https://www.ncbi.nlm.nih.gov /pubmed/27126575.

Wild Fatty Fish

In addition to being a source of protein, fatty fish such as wild salmon (if you choose canned salmon, look for "Wild Alaskan" on the label) contains omega-3 fatty acids as well. The omega-3 fats found in these types of salmon contain exceptional amounts of the vital DHA and EPA which are the long-chain omega-3s known for being most beneficial for eye, brain, and heart health. In addition to their omega-3 fats, wild salmon contain high amounts of vitamin D which can be difficult to find in most foods. Another fatty fish that you can get both fresh and canned, mackerel has even lower mercury levels and is at less risk for being over-fished.

2   M. Singh, "Essential fatty acids, DHA and human brain.," NCBI, March 01, 2005, accessed September 05, 2017, https://www.ncbi.nlm.nih.gov/pubmed/15812120.

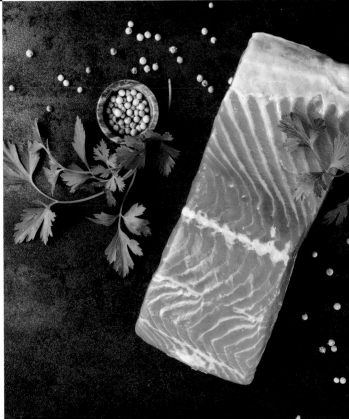

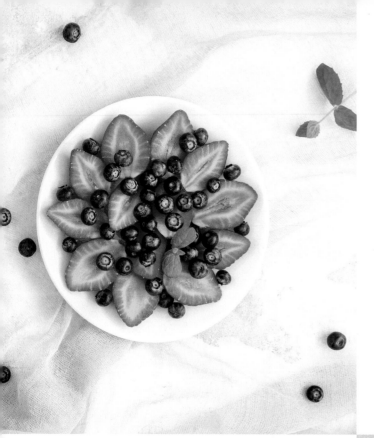

Extremely Low-Sugar Fruits

You can fit a little bit of low-sugar fruit in your keto regimen, but keep in mind your carbohydrate intake should not exceed more than 5 percent of your calories and many of your allotted carbohydrates will be dedicated to green vegetables. The lowest sugar fruits are tomato, red bell pepper, olives, and avocado. Olives and avocado are the highest in fat so those can be consumed much more frequently. Berries are allowed on your plan but since they are higher in sugar, those will need to be monitored more closely as too many berries can easily make you exceed your 5 percent carbohydrate limit. Low-sugar fruits do offer essential vitamins, minerals, and fiber, so we definitely recommend eating them, but in true moderation.

Grass-Fed, Organic Red Meat and Organic Poultry

Due to environmental toxins found in many animal proteins, it is ideal to consume organic and/or grass-fed selections if possible (if you consume meat and poultry). When beef, lamb, and venison are grass-fed, the composition of the meat changes, reflecting an omega-3 fatty acid profile that is more similar to wild salmon. These essential fats contain Docosahexaenoic Acid (DHA) Eicosapentaenoic Acid (EPA). DHA is critical for brain and eye health as it accounts for 40 percent of the polyunsaturated fatty acids found in the brain, and 60 percent found in the retina. Both DHA and EPA are associated with heart and cellular health, as well as lower levels of inflammation. Poultry such as organic turkey and chicken provide B vitamins, iron, zinc, potassium, and phosphorus.

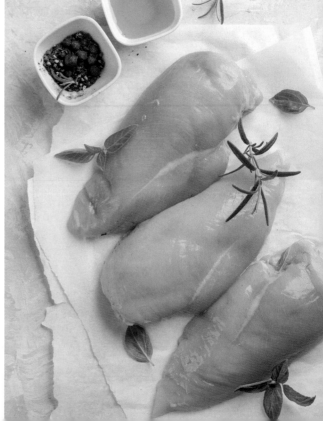

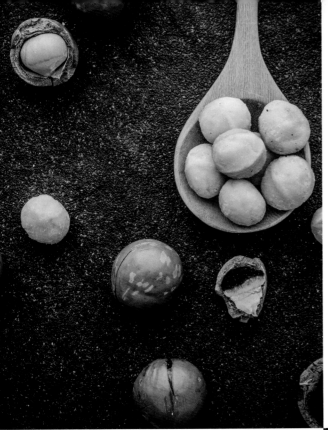

Nuts and Seeds

Nuts and seeds are packed with nutrition, providing substantial amounts of good fats, fiber, vitamins, and minerals. Aim to consume a variety of raw nuts and seeds to benefit from a broad spectrum of micronutrients. The nuts and seeds that will pack in the fat without a lot of carbohydrate are macadamia nuts, Brazil nuts, and pecans. Being calorie-dense, just 1 ounce will do as a snack or a salad topping!

Low-Carbohydrate Probiotic Foods

We all have "good" and "bad" bacteria in our bodies. Probiotics are known as the "friendly bacteria" and consist of Lactobacillus acidophilus, Lactobacillus bulgarius, Lactobacillus reuteri, Streptococcus thermophiles, Saccharomyces boulardii, Bifidobacterium bifidum, and Bacillus subtilis. Bad gut bacteria can increase for a variety of reasons (i.e., use of antibiotics, too much alcohol consumption, lack of physical movement, and smoking) so consumption of good bacteria via probiotics is beneficial. Foods that naturally contain probiotics are Greek yogurt, kefir, apple cider vinegar, low-sugar kombucha, dark chocolate, and brine-cured olives. Known as a superior probiotic food, sauerkraut actually does not contain a substantially diverse amount of friendly bacteria, however, its organic acid content supports the growth of good bacteria.

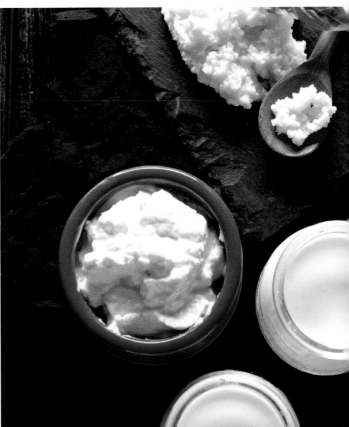

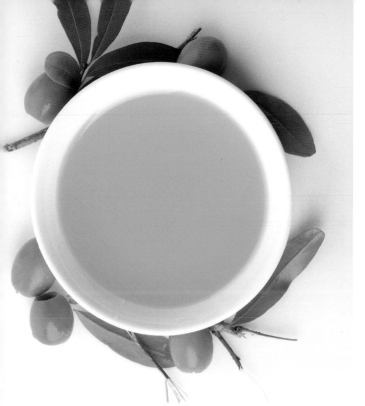

Oils

Oils are a staple to the keto diet. However, not all oils are created equally so
choosing the highest quality oils with the
most beneficial fat profiles is imperative.
In addition, the processing of some oils
(such as the use of the neurotoxin hex-
ane for extraction) can have detrimental
effects on the quality of the oil, so that is
another factor to consider. Some of the
best oils for keto, based on fat content
and cold-pressed processing, are avocado
oil, extra-virgin olive oil, coconut oil, and
walnut oil.

Water

Although it's not a food, water does get a spot
on "The Perfect 10" as its importance is unde-
niable. One of the key staples to maintaining
proper weight and health is to make good old
H_2O your primary beverage as it is sugar-
and calorie-free. Water assists with dissolving
vitamins and minerals, making them more
accessible to the body. Also, adequate water
intake is essential for the kidneys to function
which will assist with the excretion of waste
products.

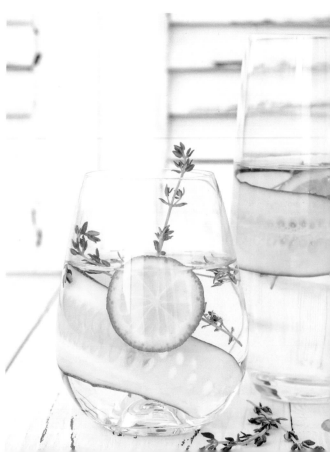

Using the Perfect 10 as your "almost keto" foundation, and avoiding the unapproved keto foods list, is all you need to do to get results, if you're uncertain about fully committing to the keto lifestyle. The most super simple way is to stick to these foods—you do not have to track your macros (carbohydrates, proteins, fats) as your lower-carbohydrate, lower-sugar meal plan will naturally fall into place by only consuming these foods. Also, feel free to choose from any listed foods found in chapter 2 for more variety, as they are all keto-approved.

Lazy Keto

Another popular route to take if one does not want to adhere to the keto macronutrient requirements is a tactic coined as "lazy keto." Lazy keto dieters only track their carbohydrates and nothing else, so if you're someone who would like one guideline to follow for reassurance but may find the fat requirement daunting, lazy keto could be the easiest way for you to ease into the lifestyle.

The first step is to establish your daily carbohydrate limit. Typically, lazy keto followers consume a maximum of 25 net carbohydrates (grams of total carbohydrates minus grams of fiber) or a maximum of 50 grams of total carbohydrates per day. All you need to do is stick to either of those carbohydrate maximums—no need to count your fat or protein intake. Of course, you will still need to eliminate the foods that are not keto-approved in order to achieve this, so sticking to the Perfect 10 foods will help you achieve the lazy keto protocol.

Almost Keto and Lazy Keto are two of the best ways to ease into keto if you're not ready to fully commit. And keep in mind, both strategies are highly effective and produce dramatic results so it isn't necessarily required to advance to the standard ketogenic nutrition plan. If you're content with loosely following the keto lifestyle and you're seeing results, you can remain in these stages. Or you can use either of these middle grounds as a stepping-stone to fully advance into the ketogenic lifestyle.

Chapter 9

Twenty of the Most Common Keto Questions, Answered

I f you have questions about what you have read so far, you will probably find the answers in this chapter. Essentially, you can consider the answers to these questions as rules to follow while following the keto protocol. Some of the "rules" may seem strict at first but your body will adjust, you will see incredible results, and your relationship with food will make a drastic change. Those who adopt the keto lifestyle realize they may have previously been consuming excessive amounts of sugar, carbohydrates, and processed foods. Improvements in how you feel and the noticeable changes in your body will convince you to not resort back to the standard American diet of excessive amounts of sugar, breads, pastas, cereals, crackers, and processed foods. These rules are in place to help take the guesswork out of your eating plan, and you will also find solutions to common roadblocks.

In a quick summary, what can and can't I eat on my keto plan?

You can eat low-carbohydrate vegetables, extremely low-sugar fruits, seafood, meat, poultry, eggs, cheese, cottage cheese, Greek yogurt, cream, butter, ghee, nuts, seeds, oils, dark chocolate, and keto-approved condiments such as mayonnaise, dressings, and sauces. You cannot consume bread, cereal, pasta, rice, crackers, potatoes, low-fat dairy, moderate- or high-carbohydrate fruits and vegetables, starches, sugary foods, soda, fruit juice, and typical dessert foods.

What are macronutrients and why are they important to know about?

Fats, carbohydrates, and proteins are the three macronutrients found in the diet. For keto, fat intake should be between 70 and 80 percent of total calories, carbohydrate intake should be between 5 and 10 percent of total calories, and protein should be between 10 and 20 percent of total calories.

How many grams of carbohydrates should I have per day?

This is a tricky question since we are all different so carbohydrate amounts will vary from person to person. Generally speaking, you should stick to 50 grams of total carbohydrates or less per day, or 25 grams of net carbohydrates (total carbohydrates minus grams of fiber) or less per day.

How do I track all of my carbohydrates, fats, and proteins?

There are many online macro tracking apps that are simple to use—one of the most popular ones in the keto community is called Carb Manager. If you're worried about this being too much work, it will only last two to three weeks before you are naturally accustomed to knowing what foods have the proper amount of carbohydrates, fats, and proteins for your nutrition plan. Although this process may seem daunting in the beginning, it gets extremely easy and then before you know it, you won't need to track anymore as you will know what is in most foods.

Do I need to track my calories, too?

People of different heights, weights, ages, activity levels, and goals all have assorted calorie requirements. Not to mention, when it comes to weight loss, calories in versus calories expended will always matter to some degree. Even if you hit your macro requirements in perfect ranges, you could still fail to lose weight (or even gain weight) if you overeat too many calories. There are several online tools to help you determine how many calories you should consume to maintain or lose weight.

Will the keto diet make my cholesterol worse since it's high in fat?

One of the primary guidelines of *Super Simple Keto* is to choose the healthiest fats possible. Fats found in foods such as avocado, extra-virgin olive oil, nuts, seeds, and wild salmon actually help to promote good cholesterol. If one focuses on unhealthy fats such as inferior oils and processed meats, then it is possible that negative outcomes such as increased bad cholesterol and excessive sodium levels could occur. There are several studies which show that the ketogenic nutrition plan is associated with improvements in good cholesterol, cardiovascular risk, and type 2 diabetes.[1]

Will I get enough fiber and micronutrients?

If your 5 to 10 percent allotted carbohydrates are dedicated to mostly green vegetables and low-sugar fruits, you can get the required fiber, vitamin, and mineral intake. The average American only consumes 10 to 15 grams of fiber per day so if you plan correctly, you can double the amount of fiber that the average person gets if you watch what you eat. The table below illustrates one example (there are several other combinations in which you can achieve this with different produce) of how you can get 24 grams of fiber while remaining under your limit of 25 grams of net carbohydrates. Not to mention, the consumption of this many servings of low-sugar produce will give a substantial amount of essential vitamins, minerals, and antioxidants.

Food	Net Carbohydrates (grams)	Fiber (grams)
1 cup cooked spinach	2 grams	4 grams
2 cups chopped romaine lettuce	1 gram	2 grams
2 cups cooked broccoli	12 grams	10 grams
½ cup raspberries	7 grams	8 grams
Totals	**22 grams**	**24 grams**

Will I have to spend a lot of time cooking?

Typically speaking, some cooking and food preparation does come along with the territory of living a healthy lifestyle. To follow keto, you will need to spend an average of three hours per week (or twenty-five minutes per day) in the kitchen to execute your eating

---

1   Kosinski, Christophe, and François R Jornayvaz. "Effects of Ketogenic Diets on Cardiovascular Risk Factors: Evidence from Animal and Human Studies." Nutrients. MDPI, May 19, 2017. https://www.ncbi.nlm.nih.gov/pmc/articles/PMC5452247/.

plan. Of course, it could be done in less time if you dine in restaurants frequently (refer to chapters 14 and 15 for your guides to restaurant and fast food keto).

So, I can eat in restaurants? Can I do that often?

Yes, you can! Some who are looking to lose weight or improve health are reluctant to even try a keto nutrition plan as they assume restaurants will be off limits. Let's face it, a large percentage of the population eat in restaurants on a regular basis due to work obligations, social gatherings, and just for plain convenience. We have dedicated chapter 14 for those who fall into this category. You will find several examples of typical restaurant scenarios and how to modify your meals to make them keto.

Can I get fast food too?

We are looking to optimize health and wellness (in addition to achieving weight loss) so while you can eat in restaurants fairly often, we will suggest minimizing fast food intake. Reason being, fast food consists of inferior ingredients and detrimental additives. Of course, if you're in a pinch and fast food is the only option, refer to chapter 15 for a list of the most popular fast food chains and how to order keto meals at each of them.

I always eat things like sandwiches and cereal—what will I replace those items with?

There are plenty of common mainstream foods that are a part of many standard diets, but they are not allowed on the keto nutrition plan due to higher carbohydrate and sugar content. This table of simple keto food swaps on the next page will help you navigate the best and tastiest substitutions.

Instead of This	Have This
Cheeseburger on a bun	Cheeseburger on a plate by itself or wrapped in lettuce
Sandwich on bread	Sandwich fillings wrapped in lettuce or over a bed of greens
Chicken pasta dish	Chicken with riced cauliflower or zucchini noodles and sauce
Steak with potatoes	Steak with vegetables or salad
Sugary salad with cranberries, candied nuts, and sweet dressing	Salad with nuts, cheese, avocado, protein, and savory oil-based dressing
Sides like French fries, rice, potato, bread, or pasta	Extra vegetables topped with butter or oil, mashed or riced cauliflower, small side salad topped with oil-based dressing
Chicken fingers or other breaded proteins with ketchup	Grilled chicken or other grilled proteins with creamy dipping sauce such as avocado oil mayo
Tacos in tortillas	Lettuce wrapped tacos
Burritos in tortillas	Burrito bowls with protein, vegetables, cheese, avocado, sour cream, and salsa
Piece of toast with peanut butter	Celery sticks with peanut butter
Ice cream	Berries topped with heavy whipping cream
Bread basket	Charcuterie board with cheese, meats, olives, and nuts
Dessert of cookies or baked goods	Red wine with dark chocolate and cheese
Standard breakfast with omelet, bacon, potatoes, and toast	Omelet with cheese, bacon, and sliced tomatoes or berries
Sweetened coffee beverage	Unsweetened coffee with coconut oil, cream, butter, or MCT oil
Salted chips	Salted nuts

Can I eat any sort of fat to fulfill my 70 to 80 percent fat requirement?

We urge against a "free-for-all" of consuming any and all fats just for the sake of fulfilling your macronutrient quotas. Most people do not consume enough omega-3 fatty acids because only certain foods contain them. Omega-3 fats are not produced by our bodies so we need to get them from our diet; they assist with brain function, heart health, and reducing inflammation. Good fats also help our blood sugar levels remain even and they can help us feel full for longer. Some examples of foods that have the healthiest fats are oysters, egg yolks, salmon, mackerel, grass-fed beef, avocado oil, olive oil, walnuts, macadamia nuts, chia seeds, and avocado.

Can I use artificial sweeteners or keto-approved sweeteners?

As nutritionists, we really want you to kick the sugar habit and that means training your taste buds (yes, they are trainable!) to not feel the need to sweeten food and drinks. This can be difficult as the standard American diet tends to make us sugar-addicted, but it is possible to break the habit and ridding sugar and sugar substitutes from your life for at least thirty days will help make the transition to living a lower-sugar lifestyle. If you feel that adding some sugar substitutes will make the keto transition easier, refer to chapter 11 to learn about the different options and what may be best for you.

Do I have to pack my food?

Packing a healthy lunch or at least some healthy snacks to have around the office or at school is one of the most efficient ways to combat workplace donuts and vending machines because if you're not hungry, passing up the treats is far easier. We don't want you spending hours in your kitchen, so if you're unsure of how to quickly prepare lunches and snacks to last you through the week, please refer to chapter 12 to learn the art of "batch-base" cooking.

Do I have to buy organic produce, grass-fed meats and butter, and wild fish to do keto?

No, you do not. We recommend these options since they help to limit pesticides and environmental toxins, however, sometimes they are not readily available and they can be expensive. You can still adhere to your keto plan even if you choose conventional versions of these foods.

Do I have to measure ketones to make sure I'm in ketosis?

No, you are not required to do this. Some find it helpful, however, a large percentage of keto dieters do not take this extra step. You may find that you will see dramatic weight loss and blood sugar level improvements just by following the keto nutrition protocol as your sugar and carbohydrate intake will be drastically cut. That alone is typically effective for results.

If I cave in and eat something sugary or with lots of carbohydrates, do I have to quit and start over?

No! Jump back on that wagon immediately! Many popular diets require one to start over if a piece (or even a bite) of cake at a birthday party occurs. This train of thought can lead to reluctance, and even anxiety when it comes to taking the first step to making a lifestyle change. There is misconception that proper nutrition has to be followed 100 percent of the time, and there is no wiggle room if you want to see results, but that can't be further from the truth. You will see progress (and lots of it) if you adhere to the keto principles and strategies most of the time. There may be situations when a slip-up occurs—acknowledge it, don't feel guilty about it, and jump right back on the wagon.

Can I use processed and packaged foods that say they are keto-approved?

Super Simple Keto urges against regular use of processed foods—it's a reset to give perspective on how many of these items we may have been consuming in the past. Not to mention, keto processed food marketing makes not-so-virtuous foods appear as falsely healthy and keto-approved. Regular use of these packaged items can certainly sabotage your goals as the macronutrient content tends to be exaggerated in terms of being low in net carbohydrates by using "fake fibers" which our bodies don't process in the same way as fiber found in foods like green vegetables. To learn more about these keto processed foods and how they may sabotage your results, refer to chapter 11.

Can I ever eat a non-keto food?

The short answer is yes, but this really depends on individual preferences. In theory, if you were extremely low in carbohydrates all day and then wanted one serving of a non-keto food that was higher in carbohydrates, you could still fall into your daily guideline of carbohydrates. Or if you aren't concerned with constantly remaining in ketosis then having a cheat won't make a huge difference as long as you jump back on the wagon. On the flip side, if you are in ketosis regularly and that's important to you, a cheat food can kick you out of ketosis (and possibly make you feel a little sick). Getting back into ketosis could take a few days.

What do I do after I hit my weight loss goal? Do I have to stay keto forever?

There are no long-term studies (more than six months) for the ketogenic diet so we don't recommend being keto indefinitely, although many keto dieters do and their anecdotal health outcomes are positive. Referring back to chapter 8, we talked about the "almost keto" way of eliminating certain foods but not counting macros. Essentially, that's how you wean off as well. Still eliminate obvious non-keto foods such as grains and sugar, but you can ease up on the strict carbohydrate requirement by way of more green veggies, low-sugar fruits (and maybe even some beans/legumes). Upping your carbohydrate intake will naturally lower your fat intake.

The ketogenic diet can seem daunting and hard to understand—we hope this Q and A chapter has cleared up any confusion. Like any nutrition lifestyle, once you sort out the facts and get into a routine, you'll find that keto is pretty simple. Once you complete your first thirty days of *Super Simple Keto*, you'll be so well-versed that the days of tracking macronutrients or searching for questions and answers will be over!

Chapter 10

Super Simple
Tactics for Success

Now that you know all about the keto diet, we would like to provide you with some additional tactics for success. Some of these address topics of food intake, while others talk about mental aspects of nutrition and weight loss. In addition, you will find pointers with regard to specific situations where sticking to a food regimen may be more difficult, and ways to overcome nutrition plan slip-ups (which happen to everyone!).

Tactic (1) Find the Way that Works for You

Some want to jump right into keto and/or ketosis immediately to get the fastest results possible, while others are a bit more hesitant to commit (refer to chapter 8 and learn about "almost keto" if this is you). Wherever you fall on the spectrum of keto readiness, adopt a routine that works for you. If keto seems far too strict for your preferences, you will still find results in the "almost keto" approach and it will allow you to work slowly but steadily up to full-blown keto.

Tactic (2) Take It Day by Day

Let's say you want to dive right into standard keto but you have a hard-to-kick soda habit that you want to try to give up cold turkey. If you think in terms of months or weeks or even several days, that can sound overwhelming and maybe even impossible. Take it one day at a time and set a goal for the day. When a goal is very short-term (such as 24 hours) it's far easier to reach and it isn't as daunting as thinking long-term.

Tactic ③ Wean Off a Bad Habit Slowly

If you can't give up your vice of choice right off the bat, that's totally fine—not many people can! Try weaning off gradually in an attempt to create new habits. Let's get back to the soda as an example since that obstacle is common for so many would-be keto dieters. If you drink three sodas per day, simply start by only drinking two sodas per day. That way, the change can be less jarring as it will happen gradually. After a couple of weeks of two sodas, try to get to one soda or even one and a half. After a month or two, maybe you can attempt the day-by-day task of zero sodas! Slowly eliminating non-keto foods will surely lead you to the point where you can eventually go full keto.

Tactic ④ Find Other Activities to Fill Your Time

It's all too common to eat when not even hungry—usually boredom, sadness, or stress tend to be the main triggers. Finding activities to solve boredom or to use as a coping mechanism can replace the emotional need for food. Taking a walk or jog, getting some errands or household tasks out of the way, relaxing in a bubble bath, finding a good book, or taking up a new hobby are simple ways to replace food as a "thing to do." Physical activity can be the most efficient as exercise gets the blood pumping and endorphins flowing, causing the feelings of hunger (i.e., sugar cravings) to subside.

Tactic ⑤ Find Substitutions that Give Satisfaction

Evaluate exactly what you like about a non-keto food and try to replicate some of those favorite tastes with keto-approved foods. For example, you may love potato chips just for the salty taste, so it's possible that other salty foods such as nuts or olives may do the trick. Or if it's the crunch that you enjoy from chips and guacamole, some crisp celery or jicama dipped in mashed avocado will satisfy the same craving. Pasta can be hard for some to give up but let's face it, the sauce is usually the flavorful addition that we love about pasta. Try using Alfredo sauce without the noodles—it makes a creamy addition to chicken or zucchini. Nighttime can be hard for those with a sweet tooth—some dark chocolate and a glass of red wine is a keto treat that may subside the craving. You can find more substitution ideas on page 66.

Tactic (6) Reward Yourself

Some bad nutrition habits are expensive! Let's take alcohol, for example. Happy hour or even some wine at home with dinner certainly adds up. If you abstain from the habit, add up the amount of money you have saved and get yourself something special. Not only will your waistline improve, but you'll also enjoy some new clothes or a gadget with all that money you saved.

Tactic (7) Take Charge of Your Social Group

Does your friend group eat out a lot? If so, take charge of *where* your friend group eats, confirming there are healthy choices for you to enjoy as well. Does your friend group drink a lot? If so, plan other social activities that involve physical activity or the outdoors. Explore new options around your area! Also, you may be surprised to find that your friends are interested in adopting new habits as well, so they may pleasantly welcome the change and suggestions.

Tactic (8) Make a Statement

Make sure you are open by sharing with your friends and family about your journey and the changes you are implementing. With regard to celebrations, you can still participate; however, take the initiative and bring approved foods such as veggie platters to parties so there is a healthier option. Suggest other home-cooked meals or snacks for others to bring to the party as well! Just as with Tactic 7, being vocal about your goals and newfound lifestyle may inspire others to join you, and it's always more fun to have a buddy.

Tactic ⑨ Eat Consciously

If you don't want to count calories and macros (it's definitely not required!), a good rule of thumb to follow is to listen to your body and eat consciously. Eating consciously means eating when you are hungry and stopping when you are 80 percent full. It is easier said than done sometimes but when we eat consciously, we avoid eating out of boredom, stress, or social pressure. Also, it is best to provide focus on your food instead of allocating attention to a book or movie since many tend to overeat while their minds are occupied by something else. If you prefer not to count your calories and macros, that is perfectly fine, but it can be useful to employ the "Seven Scales of Hunger" and try to always hover around level four.

Seven Scales of Hunger

7. **About to burst:** Ate way too much food but it was fun! Same feeling you may experience after Thanksgiving dinner or a birthday party and you think you may never want to see food again.

6. **Extremely full:** Feeling some discomfort/bloat and need to lie down.

5. **Pretty full:** Had a few extra bites after being satiated and won't need to eat again for some time.

4. **Comfortably satisfied:** Ate for fullness and not just for fun or out of boredom; stopped when 80% full (this is easiest to attain when you eat slowly so your brain has time to signal to your stomach).

3. **A tad bit uncomfortable:** Didn't eat quite enough (around 70% full) and feel a snack (or more) is needed in the near future.

2. **Uncomfortable:** May have the "growling" sensation in the stomach and or experience low energy.

1. **Miserable:** Extremely low on energy, unable to focus on tasks, and possibly irritable.

Tactic ⑩ Control Calories and Portions

Like we have mentioned, counting calories is not required; however, it can be beneficial to have a general idea of how many calories is right for you and your goals, since many people eat far more calories than their bodies need. Despite the fact that the main purpose of food is to fuel our bodies, it is commonly used for comfort, fun, social purposes, and as a solution to boredom. Eating proper portions and not until you feel "stuffed" is a key component to achieving and maintaining your ideal weight. The average American is told to consume 2,000 calories per day but this figure is completely wrong for millions of people. For example, if you are a woman who is 5'4" and want to weigh 125 pounds, your required intake will range anywhere from 1400–1800 calories per day depending on age and activity level.

Tactic (11) Stick to Your Grocery List and Never Shop While Hungry

Before leaving for the grocery store, make a list and stick to it during your shopping trip. If you don't buy junk food and have it around the house, you are much less likely to eat junk food. The foods found in chapter 2 are all allowed in the shopping cart, but of course, you don't need to purchase all of them—start with your favorites. Always remember to avoid a hungry trip to the grocery store as non-keto foods or extra foods in general may end up in the cart.

Tactic (12) Be Prepared at Work

The workplace is typically a junk food haven. Office donuts, cookies, chips, sodas, and candy vending machines are incredibly tempting, especially when you're hungry. Not to mention, unhealthy snacking may be the norm in your office so the "everybody's doing it" attitude adds to the temptation of giving in. Not being hungry can be the most effective way of combating the weight gaining food that's in your workplace. It only takes five minutes to put together a convenient snack pack that will keep your hunger satiated and blood sugar levels even. It's as easy as putting a few healthy snacks in your bag the night before work—items like hard boiled eggs, raw nuts, vegetables and mashed avocado, Greek yogurt, berries, and healthy dinner leftovers.

Tactic (13) Healthy Restaurant Choices

You can still achieve your goals while dining out! If you have a hectic work schedule or you just enjoy eating in restaurants, try to employ the following key concepts when eating in restaurants. For a photo guide of exactly what to eat when dining out, refer to chapter 14.

- Skip the breadbasket—even if it's put in front of you, kindly ask the server to take it away.
- Replace rice, potato, and pasta side dishes with vegetables.
- Use plain oil and vinegar for salad dressing.
- Eliminate pasta and bread-based dishes such as pizza, burgers, and sandwiches; if you order a sandwich or burger, ask your server to lettuce wrap it (most restaurants will oblige).
- Ask what's in the soup—some have grain-based fillers that you'll want to avoid. Stick to ones made with cream, butter, or avocado bases.
- Ask for any sauces on the side and try to use sparingly.
- Order fresh berries with heavy cream for dessert.
- Avoid waffles, French toast, pancakes, donuts, pastries, or hash browns at breakfast, and opt for egg-based dishes. Keep in mind, any benedict can be made with sliced tomatoes as the base, instead of bread!
- If a restaurant meal is huge (and they usually are), take half of it home and have it for lunch the next day.
- National restaurant chains are required to have nutrition information on site. Check it out—it may save you a thousand calories!

Tactic (14) Watch Out for Drinkable Sugar

A fruit juice with breakfast, Starbucks Frappuccino in the afternoon, and one soda at dinner add up to almost 900 calories and 100 grams of sugar! People can tend to ignore liquid calories and don't realize how easily they compile and result in weight gain. The habit of drinking water is a key staple to losing weight and achieving wellness. Unfortunately, soda and fruit juice have around the same amounts of calories, carbohydrates, and sugar. Even though fruit juice has natural sugar, it's still sugar and sugar turns into fat if it isn't burned. If you're looking for a good source of Vitamin C without the added sugar, opt for items like broccoli, bell pepper, Brussels sprouts, or raspberries.

Tactic (15) Step Off the Wagon—Don't Fall

If you maintain balanced nutrition on a regular basis, then splurging occasionally will not hurt your weight loss goals as long as you return to your good habits immediately after the splurge. Also, if you plan your splurges ahead of time, you will be nutritionally prepared to afford your treat. If you know you're going to a restaurant on Friday night that has your favorite chocolate torte then be sure to stick to your nutrition plan on Monday, Tuesday, Wednesday, and Thursday, and enjoy your night out on Friday. Once Saturday morning arrives, do not have the "I ruined everything last night so who cares what I eat today" attitude. Another key concept of weight loss is getting right back on the wagon after taking a controlled step off it.

Tactic (16) Avoid "Train Gain"

If you enjoy exercise, avoid the big mistake of overeating—you will still gain weight, despite the fact you are working out. The average person's workout will only burn around 500 calories so it is imperative to stick to your nutrition regimen after an exercise session. Too many caloric rewards for a job well done at the gym will backfire and negate all of the hard work you have put in.

We have all heard that people who work out need to "carb up" and eat more calories to have enough energy. This may be true for extremely competitive Ironman triathletes or Olympic athletes but if you're working out like a typical person (jogging eight miles per week or spending six hours per week in the gym), there is no physical need to store away excess carbohydrates to be used for energy. Keep in mind, to lose one pound of weight per week, you must cut out 500 calories from your daily intake. If you spend an hour exercising, you can reach this 500-calorie deficit and your work is done for the day. If you return home from the gym and reward yourself with four slices of pizza (1300 calories) instead of a sensible 600-calorie meal, you are now in excess of 800 calories. Not working out? Replace a morning scone with two eggs and some blueberries, and an afternoon soda with unsweetened iced tea and there's your 500-calorie deficit!

Tactic (17) Don't Feel Obligated to Exercise to Make a Lifestyle Change

When it comes to weight loss and health improvements, you need to pick and choose your battles. For some, the thought of heading to the gym at 5:00 a.m. before a long day of work prevents many from ever attempting to make a healthy lifestyle change. Fortunately, weight loss and blood sugar improvements are primarily based on good nutrition—working out merely fine-tunes the effort one puts into his or her daily nutrition plan. If the thought of working out is holding you back from making a change, know that you are not required to add exercise to achieve significant results.

Tactic (18) Keep it Simple

Keto can seem complicated and overwhelming but it's just a matter of focusing on a few simple concepts. If you take these seven steps and implement them into your daily routine, weight loss and wellness will happen for you!

1. Stick to your keto macros—70 to 80 percent fat, 10 to 20 percent protein, and 5 to 10 percent carbohydrates.
2. Focus on nutrient-dense whole foods, not on keto processed foods.
3. Eat healthy fats and high-quality proteins.
4. Use green vegetables and low sugar fruits as a primary carbohydrate and fiber source.
5. Eliminate non-keto foods such as grains and sugars.
6. Exercise if possible (but it is not required).
7. Make a plan, prepare, and stick to the guidelines.

Chapter 11

What You Need to Know about Processed Keto Foods

Keto is one of most popular diet trends in recent years, so of course the processed food industry has used this opportunity to take advantage of and capitalize on unknowing consumers. You will find thousands of "keto" processed food products marketed as convenient while fitting in the guidelines of the low-carbohydrate protocol. Two of the most frequently used tag lines on packaging are "zero net carbs" and "sugar-free," but unfortunately, if we delve into the science behind these statements, you'll find that these foods could sabotage your goals.

Net Carbohydrates in Processed Foods

As explained previously, keto dieters gauge their carbohydrate intake by total carbohydrates or net carbohydrates. Total carbohydrates are listed as all carbohydrates found on the nutrition label (usually, people stick to 50 grams or less per day) and net carbohydrates are counted as total carbohydrates minus fiber (since fiber cannot be digested and essentially, doesn't "count" towards

Ingredients

Modified wheat starch
Water
Wheat gluten
Wheat protein isolate
Oat fiber
(Chicory) vegetable fiber
Wheat bran
Soybean oil
Yeast
Vinegar
Salt
Calcium propionate
Sorbic acid

Nutrition Facts

Serving Size: 1 Slice
Calories: 45
Fat: 1 gram
Saturated fat: 0 grams
Cholesterol: 0 milligrams
Sodium: 75 milligrams
Carbohydrates: 9 grams
Dietary Fiber: 9 grams
Sugars: 0 grams
Protein: 5 grams

the total carbohydrate amount)—usually, people stick to 25 grams of net carbohydrates or less per day.

Why do we subtract fiber from total carbohydrates to calculate "net carbs"? The short answer is because fiber is a nondigestible carbohydrate so we really can't process it, so therefore it does not affect the blood sugar. Unfortunately, the fiber used in most keto processed foods is not the same as the fiber found in green vegetables, so it can affect our systems in a completely different manner. Let's explore a popular processed keto bread which is marketed as "zero net carbs."

At first glance of the ingredients list and nutrition facts, you may be wondering how a product packed with wheat and oats can be keto-friendly, and even more questionable, have zero net carbohydrates. If you take the 9 grams of total carbohydrates per slice, you magically get to subtract the 9 grams of fiber to get to "zero net carbs." Now, the fiber added to this bread comes from chicory root and many nutrition circles label this as a "fraudulent fiber" as it has not been shown to provide the same health benefits as true fiber found in a food like green vegetables. Inulin-containing chicory root is indigestible, so in technical terms, it can be classified as dietary fiber. The problem is it hasn't been proven to boast the same swelling property and stomach-filling effect that we experience when eating fiber-rich whole foods such as broccoli, raspberries, and avocados.

It is becoming very common for the processed food industry to add these isolated fibers such as chicory root with the intention of marketing to keto dieters. The fine, powdery consistency of these "fibers" allows food manufacturers to use them as they do not affect taste or texture. Ratcheting up the content of fiber on nutrition labels results in the allowed use of the word "fiber" and phrase "zero net carbs" on the front packaging, despite the fact that the used fiber may come from "fraudulent fiber" sources that do not have the same benefits as the traditional dietary fiber. Look for the following ingredients to spot possible fraudulent fiber in processed foods.

Fiber (IMO)
IMO Fiber (Powder or Syrup)
Prebiotic Fiber
VitaFiber
Inulin
Chicory root

Net Carbohydrates Calculated by Subtracting Fiber and Sugar Alcohols

Many keto circles advise to calculate net carbo-hydrates as total carbohydrates minus fiber and sugar alcohols. Sugar alcohols are a hybrid of sugar and alcohol molecules but do not contain ethanol (the compound that causes intoxication) and are categorized as sweet carbohydrates. They are not calorie-free although they do have less cal-ories than sugar, and they do activate the tongue's sweet receptors so they are used to sweeten foods. Some keto circles recommend subtracting these sugar alcohols (in addition to fiber) to get your net carbohydrate count because sugar alcohols affect the blood sugar less than regular sugar, and due to the fact they are not fully digestible. The reason why we have not advised to calculate net carbohydrates this way is because it could possibly sabotage your goals.

Common Types of Sugar Alcohols

Modified wheat starch
Erythritol
Xylitol
Sorbitol
Maltitol
Mannitol
Isomalt
Lactitol
Hydrogenated starch hydrolysates

Sugar alcohol is a carbohydrate so even though its impact on blood sugar is less than that of real sugar, it can still raise blood sugar levels if you eat too much of it. Since sugar alcohols are hard to absorb, they will affect you less than regular sugar but they are not entirely a free pass. It is common for many keto dieters to subtract all grams of sugar alcohols from the total carbohydrate amount on a food label. Since sugar alcohols still have some effect on blood sugar, we advise to only subtract half the amount of sugar alcohols from total carbohydrates to get your net carbohydrate amount. For example, if a keto packaged food has 25 grams of total carbohydrates and 20 grams of sugar alco-hols, you would take half of the grams of sugar alcohols and subtract that from the total carbohydrates.

25 (total carbs) - 10 (sugar alcohols) = 15 grams of net carbohydrates

You will see that using this more accurate formula may cause you to determine that the net carbohydrate count is far too high to consume many (or any) servings of the particular keto processed food. Essentially, you should treat sugar alcohols in a similar fashion as sugar and limit your intake as the progress of thousands of keto dieters has stalled due to regular consumption of these sweeteners. Not to mention, sugar alcohols have also been shown to produce side effects such as gas, bloating, and abdominal discomfort since they are only partially digested. (However, erythritol is usually better tolerated, if you're concerned about these side effects.) As with most situations, if something seems too good to be true (like eating as much "zero carb" ice cream as you like) then it probably is.

Artificial Sweeteners

Artificial sweeteners add sweetness to foods without adding any calories. Some keto circles approve the use of Aspartame (Equal or NutraSweet), Acesulfame Potassium (Sunett), or Sucralose (Splenda) to give more flavor without impacting weight gain or blood sugar levels. Studies are now suggesting that regular consumption of artificial sweeteners in the general population is actually associated with negative health outcomes such as type 2 diabetes and metabolic disorders, as opposed to helping prevent them.[1] One 2016 study showed that normal-weight adults who consumed more artificial sweeteners were more likely to have diabetes than people who were overweight or obese. Another 2014 study exhibited that these sweeteners, such as saccharin, can alter the composition of gut bacteria. This change can result in glucose intolerance, which is the initial step towards metabolic syndrome and diabetes. Not to mention, certain artificial sweeteners such as aspartame are associated with cancer risks due carcinogenic properties.[2] The bottom line is your body responds to artificial sweeteners differently than it

---

1   Swithers, S. "Artificial sweeteners produce the counterintuitive effect of inducing metabolic derangements," NCBI, September 2013, accessed September 24, 2017, https://www.ncbi.nlm.nih.gov/pmc/articles/PMC3772345/.

2   Soffritti, M., M. Padovani, E. Tibalidi, L. Falcioni, F. Manservisi, and F. Belpoggi. "The Carcinogenic Effects of Aspartame: The Urgent Need for Regulatory Re-evaluation." NCBI. April 2014. Accessed April 14, 2019. https://www.ncbi.nlm.nih.gov/pubmed /24436139.

does regular sugar. Artificial sugar can interfere with innately learned taste, and this can confuse the brain, which will send signals telling you to eat even more sweetened foods.

Stevia, Swerve, and Monk fruit

Besides sugar alcohols, Stevia, Swerve, and Monk fruit are some of the most popular keto sweeteners and they are touted as more "natural" than artificial sweeteners such as aspartame. Moderate use of Stevia is approved in many keto circles as it is a zero-calorie sweetener that is derived from the plant species Stevia rebaudiana, native to Brazil and Paraguay. While stevia itself is natural, brands that include it are usually highly processed and may contain other ingredients. For example, Truvia goes through forty processing steps during manufacturing. Abundant use of these processed zero-calorie sweeteners is fairly new, and future research may shed more light on the impact of consuming them on a regular basis. Although it is easier said than done, training your taste buds to not be required to add sweeteners to beverages and foods for satisfaction is a key outcome we would like you to achieve.

A highly popular keto sweetener, Swerve is a sugar replacement made from erythritol, oligosaccharides, and "natural flavors," though it's unknown what exact sources the food manufacturer uses for said natural flavors. As previously mentioned, erythritol is a sugar alcohol; the oligosaccharides in Swerve are created by adding enzymes to starchy root vegetables. Swerve claims to be calorie-free and to have no effects on blood sugar or insulin levels; however, large quantities may cause digestive distress.

Another widely-used keto sweetener, monk fruit extract comes from the small green gourd which resembles a melon. Sometimes the extract is blended with dextrose or other ingredients in order to balance the sweet taste. Despite the fact that monk fruit extract is 150 to 200 times sweeter than sugar, it is touted to have zero calories and carbohydrates. Monk fruit gets its sweet taste from antioxidant mogrosides, and studies state the extract can be used as a low-glycemic natural sweetener.

All in all, we are not saying that you can *never* consume the ingredients listed in this chapter, although, if you are going to partake, true moderation is key. If you're really craving a keto sweet treat or you need a packaged food on-the-go here and there, limited use of these foods will not entirely sabotage your goals. We recommend no more than three servings per week of these foods due to four key reasons: limited long-term research, the potential for raised blood sugar, food manufacturing exaggerations making not-so-virtuous foods appear healthy, and the most important—training your taste buds to enjoy whole foods without added sweeteners.

Chapter 12

Super Simple Batch and Batch-Base Cooking

You've probably heard of "batch cooking" before but "batch-base cooking" may be new to you. We coined this process and term and it's our preferred super simple way to cook. First of all, if you aren't familiar with batch-cooking, let's start there for some background information.

This is a process many people employ to help get as close as possible to having ready-made healthy meals without hiring a meal service or personal chef, and this technique is called batch-cooking. Reflecting its name, batch cooking means exactly that—preparing and cooking large portions of meals all at once so you can keep extra in the freezer or fridge to simply unfreeze and/or reheat future meals. The two complaints we usually hear from batch cookers are: "I don't like reheating my dinner in a microwave, and my food (specifically salad or veggies) seems wilted or not fresh." While we enjoy batch-cooking meals such as casseroles, soups, and stews due to the fact that they come out "new" after reheating, we prefer a different technique for other meals.

To avoid these potential mishaps, we would like to illustrate the art of "batch-base cooking" and this process involves batch cooking the base of the meal which usually includes the proteins. Proteins always take the longest to prepare and they can be refrigerated and stored for longer periods of time (compared to something like salad), and they heat up nicely on the stovetop to give that home-cooked meal feel while keeping the meal preparation time at less than ten minutes.

Expedited Breakfast

Breakfast can be extremely quick and easy, so let's just knock it out at home before your day begins. There are tactics to ensure your breakfast takes no more than fifteen minutes (including prep and eating) in the morning before heading to work, school, or errands. The night before, be sure to do the following tasks that apply to you:

- Put water and coffee grounds in the coffee pot and preset.
- Or have your selected tea (or other low-carbohydrate beverage) ready to go.
- Know what you will eat the next morning (this sounds basic but making a mental plan beforehand will help you prepare).
- Take inventory on your groceries—make sure everything you need is in there.
- Set your alarm to ensure you have an extra fifteen minutes in the morning—it's a commitment but it's just fifteen extra minutes—you can do it!

Expedited Breakfast Ideas

Keto Coffee (recipe on page 177)
Plain coffee with cream, butter, or ghee
2-3 eggs your way with optional sides of tomatoes, avocado, or berries
Scrambled eggs topped with cheese, avocado, salsa
Plain yogurt (Greek, almond, coconut) topped with berries, nut butter, and hemp seeds
Chia Pudding (recipe on page 175)
Cottage cheese with berries
Breakfast charcuterie box (hard-boiled egg, celery with cream cheese, smoked salmon, nuts, berries)

Lunch Batch-Base Cooking

The super simple way to batch cook your lunches is to pick two proteins for the week. Prepare those proteins ahead of time (on Sunday, for example) and use them in a variety of ways from Monday to Friday. Below you will find three examples of batch-base lunch options to choose from and each corresponding grocery list will contain enough ingredients for five days of lunches. If you have your favorite keto-approved proteins, produce, and toppings, feel free to come up with your own batch-base creations.

Batch-Base Option One: Tuna and Chicken

Grocery List	
○ 3 cans of tuna	$6.00
○ 1 pound of chicken	$4.99
○ 1 head of lettuce	$1.50
○ 1 bunch of celery	$1.50
○ 1 jar tomatillo sauce (green sauce)	$1.99
○ 1 bell pepper (any color)	$0.79
○ 1 yellow onion	$0.79
○ 1 large tomato	$0.79
○ 1 package shredded cheese	$3.99
○ 2 avocados	$3.00
○ Mayonnaise	$1.99
○ Mustard	$1.99
Cost Per Lunch	**$5.86**

Two protein bases to batch cook:

- Chop the chicken into bite-sized pieces and pan cook in oil and your favorite seasonings over medium heat until cooked through, around 12 minutes. Divide into 2 to 3 servings and store in the refrigerator.

- Mix the 3 cans tuna with oil, mayonnaise (optional), chopped bell pepper, chopped onion, chopped celery, and mustard. Divide into 2 to 3 servings and store in the refrigerator.

Batch-base lunch options:

- Combine 1 serving of cooked chicken with 3 tablespoons of green tomatillo sauce and reheat in the microwave for 1 minute or on the stovetop on medium heat for 5 minutes. Top with shredded cheese and sliced avocado.

- Place 1 serving of cold chicken directly on a bed of chopped lettuce. Add sliced tomatoes, avocado, and diced onion. Top with oil and vinegar or your favorite low-carbohydrate, low-sugar dressing.

- Take 1 serving of cold chicken and toss with 1 to 2 tablespoons of mayo, diced onion, diced bell pepper, diced celery, and your favorite seasonings. Scoop into lettuce cups and top with sliced avocado.

- Take 1 serving of cold tuna mixture and place in a bowl. Use celery sticks to dip.

- Place 1 serving of cold tuna mixture directly on a bed of chopped lettuce. Add sliced tomatoes, avocado, and diced onion. Top with oil and vinegar or your favorite low-carbohydrate, low-sugar dressing.

Batch-Base Option Two: Egg Salad and Charcuterie

Grocery List	
○ 1 dozen eggs	$2.99
○ 1 package deli turkey	$3.99
○ 1 package salami	$2.99
○ 1 package sliced cheese	$3.99
○ 1 package nuts	$3.99
○ 1 jar petite dill pickles	$3.99
○ 1 head of lettuce	$1.50
○ 1 bunch of celery	$1.50
○ 1 bell pepper (any color)	$0.79
○ 1 yellow onion	$0.79
○ 1 large tomato	$0.79
○ 2 avocados	$3.00
○ Mayonnaise	$1.99
○ Mustard	$1.99
Cost Per Lunch	**$6.86**

One protein base to batch cook:

- Boil 6 to 8 eggs over high heat for 10 minutes. Remove from heat and run the eggs under cold water to peel. Dice the eggs and mix with 2 tablespoons of mayonnaise, 2 teaspoons of mustard, diced celery, diced bell pepper, diced onion, and your favorite seasonings. Divide into 2 to 3 servings and store in the refrigerator.

- The charcuterie (deli meats and cheese) requires no cooking, however, you will boil 2 additional eggs over high heat for 10 minutes. Run them under cold water to peel and leave whole. Store in the refrigerator.

Batch-base lunch options:

- Place 1 serving of egg salad mixture directly on a bed of chopped lettuce. Add sliced tomatoes, avocado, and diced onion. Top with oil and vinegar or your favorite low-carbohydrate, low-sugar dressing.

- Take 1 serving of egg salad mixture and scoop into lettuce cups and top with sliced avocado.

- Take 1 serving of egg salad mixture and place in a bowl. Use celery sticks to dip.

- In a sectioned lunch box, place 2 to 3 pieces of rolled up turkey, 5 to 6 pieces of salami, 2 slices of cheese, 4 to 5 mini pickles, ½ a mashed avocado, bell pepper strips for dipping, and 1 serving of nuts.

- Chop 3 to 4 slices of turkey, 4 to 5 slices of salami, 1 to 2 slices of cheese, and place over a bed of chopped lettuce. Top with sliced tomato, diced onion, two halved hard-boiled eggs, and oil and vinegar, or your favorite low-carbohydrate, low-sugar dressing.

Batch-Base Option Three: Hearty Broccoli Salad and Ground Turkey Mirepoix

Grocery List	
○ 1 large head broccoli	$1.19
○ 1 package shredded cheddar cheese	$3.99
○ 1 red onion	$0.79
○ 1 package bacon	$2.99
○ 1 package green onions	$1.19
○ 1 avocado	$1.00
○ 1 bottle mayo-based dressing (see page 250 to make your own)	$2.99
○ 1½ pounds ground turkey	$5.99
○ 1 red bell pepper	$0.79
○ 1 bunch celery	$1.50
○ 1 yellow onion	$0.79
○ 1 (32-ounce) carton chicken broth	$1.99
○ 1 jar low-sugar marinara sauce	$2.99
○ 1 large zucchini	$0.79
Cost Per Lunch	**$5.80**

Two protein bases to batch cook:

- Chop the head of broccoli into florets and place in boiling water over high heat. In the meantime, prepare a large bowl of ice water. Boil the broccoli until slightly tender, around 3 minutes. Remove with a slotted spoon and place in the ice water to stop the cooking process. Strain the broccoli with a colander and place in a large bowl, and toss with the dressing, cooked chopped bacon, chopped red and green onion, and shredded cheese to taste. Place in 2 to 3 airtight containers and refrigerate.

- To make the mirepoix, use oil to sauté the diced red bell pepper, diced celery, and diced yellow onion for 3 minutes over medium heat. Add the ground turkey and combine with the onion mixture, while breaking into little pieces until cooked through, around 8 minutes. Season to taste and divide into 2 to 3 servings and place into airtight containers and refrigerate.

Batch-base lunch options:

- Plate 1 to 2 servings of cold broccoli salad on its own, top with diced avocado right before serving.

- Pair 1 serving of broccoli salad with 1 serving of turkey mirepoix and make a platter with mashed avocado for dipping.

- Take 1 to 2 servings of turkey mirepoix and place in large bowl; add 1 to 2 cups of chicken broth (or bone broth) and reheat to make soup.

- Take 1 to 2 servings of turkey mirepoix and add low-sugar marinara sauce to taste; reheat on the stovetop or microwave. Pair with roasted zucchini slices.

Batch Dinners

Each batch dinner includes enough ingredients to make five servings that will keep well in the refrigerator for the work week. Simply choose one batch dinner and prepare ahead of time on Sunday and you will be set for Monday through Friday. Or for more variety, choose two different batch dinners and cut the ingredients in half for each. Referring back to chapter 3's *Super Simple Keto* kitchen preparation, your required keto staples are oil, butter, water, garlic (granulated or cloves), salt, and pepper—these ingredients are not counted toward the 6-ingredient maximum for each recipe.

Pizza Casserole

1 tablespoon oil, plus more for greasing
1 (14.5-ounce) can diced tomatoes
1 pound hot Italian sausage crumbles
½ cup baby Portobello mushrooms, sliced
1 tablespoon oregano
½ tablespoon garlic powder
1½ cups shredded mozzarella cheese
15 slices pepperoni

1. Preheat oven to 425°F.

2. Grease or spray a casserole dish with oil.

3. Drain the diced tomatoes and pat dry, using a paper towel.

4. Using oil, brown the sausage over medium-high heat until cooked through, around 8 minutes. Use a spatula to break up the sausage while cooking.

5. Add the sausage to the casserole dish and top with drained tomatoes and mushrooms. Season with oregano, garlic, and salt and pepper, to taste.

6. Top with mozzarella and pepperoni and bake for 10 minutes until the cheese is thoroughly melted. Let cool for 5 to 7 minutes before serving.

Cheeseburger Casserole

1 tablespoon oil
4 cups riced cauliflower
2 cups cheddar cheese, divided
¼ cup heavy cream
2 pounds ground beef
Salt and pepper, to taste
½ cup low-sugar ketchup
2 tablespoons mustard

1. Heat the oil in a large pan over medium-high heat, and add the riced cauliflower. Stir fry until the cauliflower is tender and a little browned, about 8 to 10 minutes.

2. Remove from heat and stir in half of the cheddar cheese and all of the heavy cream.

3. Transfer the mixture to a 9x13-inch casserole dish and spread evenly; set aside.

4. Preheat the oven to 400°F; meanwhile, lightly wipe down the pan and remove any bits of cauliflower. Add the ground beef and season with salt and pepper, to taste.

5. Cook the ground beef until browned, about 10 minutes, and drain if needed. Sprinkle the ground beef evenly over the cauliflower in the casserole dish.

6. Drizzle the ketchup and mustard over the ground beef, and top with the remaining cheddar cheese.

7. Bake until the casserole is hot and the cheese has melted, about 10 minutes.

Loaded Cauliflower Casserole

1 large head cauliflower, cut into small florets

2 tablespoons butter, melted

Salt and pepper, to taste

⅔ cup sour cream

¼ cup heavy cream

2 cloves garlic, minced (or ½ tablespoon garlic powder)

1½ cups shredded cheddar cheese, divided

6 tablespoons crumbled bacon, divided

¼ cup chopped green onions, divided

1. Preheat the oven to 450°F.

2. In a large bowl, toss the cauliflower florets with the melted butter. Season with salt and black pepper, to taste.

3. Transfer the cauliflower to a glass casserole dish in a single layer, and roast in the oven for 15 to 20 minutes, until crisp-tender.

4. Meanwhile, in the same bowl, whisk together the sour cream and heavy cream, until smooth. Stir in the garlic, half of the cheddar cheese, half of the bacon, and half of the green onions.

5. When the cauliflower is done roasting, take it out and leave the oven on. Add the cauliflower to the bowl and mix with the sauce.

6. Return the cauliflower mixture to the casserole dish. Top with remaining cheese and bacon bits.

7. Bake until the cheese is thoroughly melted, about 5 to 7 minutes, and top with remaining green onions.

Green Bean Casserole

2 tablespoons oil, divided

1 large white onion, chopped

1 cup mushrooms, sliced

2 pounds green beans, cut in half or roughly chopped

3 cups canned Cream of Mushroom Soup (or see recipe on page 234)

½ cup almond flour

2 tablespoons dried minced onion

1. Preheat the oven to 375°F.

2. In a skillet over medium heat, sauté the onions and mushrooms in half of the oil until lightly browned, about 8 to 10 minutes. Remove from heat.

3. Boil the green beans until slightly tender, about 4 to 5 minutes.

4. Place the cooked green beans, mushroom/onion mixture, and cream of mushroom soup into a glass or ceramic casserole dish. Stir until combined.

5. In a small bowl, combine the almond flour and dried minced onions. Stir in the other half of the oil until crumbly. Sprinkle the topping over the casserole.

6. Bake for 18 to 20 minutes, until the topping is golden.

Chicken and Broccoli Alfredo Bowls

2 tablespoons butter

¾ cup diced yellow onion

2 cloves garlic, pressed

8 ounces white mushrooms, sliced

1½ pounds chicken breasts or thighs, cubed and cooked (you can use already prepared rotisserie chicken)

3 cups broccoli florets, steamed

2 cups store-bought or homemade Creamy Alfredo Sauce (page 246)

Chopped parsley, for garnish (optional)

1. Melt the butter in a large skillet over medium heat. Add the onions, garlic, and mushrooms, and cook until the onions are translucent and the mushrooms are cooked through, around 7 minutes.

2. Add the chicken, steamed broccoli, and Alfredo sauce. Combine and simmer for 3 minutes.

3. Divide among 5 meal storage containers and refrigerate. To serve, reheat and top with chopped parsley (optional).

Cabbage Roll Casserole

1 tablespoon oil

4 cloves garlic, minced (or 1 tablespoon garlic powder)

1½ pounds ground beef

Salt and pepper, to taste

4 cups riced cauliflower

6 cups chopped, shredded cabbage (about 1 medium head)

2 tablespoons Italian seasoning

3 cups low-sugar marinara sauce

3 cups mozzarella cheese, shredded

1. Heat the oil in a large pan over medium heat. Add the garlic and cook for up to a minute, until fragrant.

2. Increase heat to medium-high and add the ground beef. Season with salt and black pepper, to taste. Cook through, breaking apart with a spatula, until browned, about 8 to 10 minutes; drain if needed.

3. Preheat the oven to 350°F.

4. In a 9x13-inch glass baking dish, combine the riced cauliflower, chopped cabbage, and Italian seasoning.

5. After the ground beef has cooked through, add it to the baking dish and stir in marinara sauce.

6. Bake for about 30 minutes, until the cabbage is crisp-tender, and top with shredded mozzarella.

7. Continue baking for about 12 to 15 minutes, until the cheese is golden brown and the cabbage is completely cooked through.

No-Tortilla Cheesy Chicken Enchiladas in Green Sauce

2 tablespoons oil

2 pounds chicken breast, chopped

12 ounces tomatillo sauce (or salsa verde)

2 cups shredded Mexican cheese blend

Avocado, sour cream, cilantro for serving (optional)

1. In a large pan over medium-high heat, heat the oil and place the chopped chicken in the pan.

2. Cook for 3 minutes and then flip the chicken pieces over with a spatula. Reduce heat to medium.

3. Continue to cook until chicken is almost cooked through, around 8 minutes, while stirring occasionally.

4. Add the tomatillo sauce and simmer for 3 more minutes.

5. Divide into 5 servings and place into airtight containers and refrigerate.

6. Divide the shredded cheese into 5 other airtight containers and refrigerate.

7. To serve, sprinkle 1 serving of cheese over 1 serving of chicken in tomatillo sauce and reheat.

8. Top with avocado, sour cream, and cilantro (optional).

White Turkey Chili

3 tablespoons oil
1 small onion, diced
3 cloves garlic, minced
1½ pounds ground turkey
  (or beef, lamb, or pork)
Your favorite seasonings,
  to taste
3 cups riced cauliflower
3 cups full-fat coconut milk
2 tablespoons mustard

1. In a large pot, heat the oil.

2. Add the onion and garlic to the oil.

3. Stir for 2 to 3 minutes and then add the ground turkey.

4. Break up with the spatula and stir constantly until crumbled.

5. Add in your favorite seasonings and riced cauliflower, and stir well.

6. Once the meat is browned add in the coconut milk and mustard, bring to a simmer, and reduce for 5 to 8 minutes, stirring often.

7. Section into 5 airtight containers and refrigerate.

8. To serve, reheat and eat on its own or top with shredded cheese, avocado, sour cream, and salsa.

Bun-less Philly Cheesesteak Platter

3 tablespoons butter
2 cups white mushrooms,
  sliced
1 cup chopped onions
1 cup chopped green bell
  pepper
Garlic powder, to taste
1½ pounds rare roast beef
  slices
Salt and pepper, to taste
10 slices provolone cheese
  (for serving)

1. In a large saucepan over medium heat, melt the butter. Add the mushrooms, onions, bell peppers, and garlic powder. Cook until the mixture is tender, around 6 to 7 minutes.

2. Cut the roast beef into 1-inch squares and add to the saucepan.

3. Toss the roast beef with the mushrooms, onions, and bell peppers for 2 minutes until heated through. Add salt and pepper, to taste.

4. Divide into 5 airtight containers and refrigerate.

5. To serve, reheat and top with 2 slices provolone cheese.

Cheesy Chicken and Broccoli Casserole

1 cup cooked riced
   cauliflower

3 tablespoons almond meal

Your favorite seasonings

2 cups chicken broth (low
   sodium)

1 cup unsweetened almond
   milk

1 pound boneless skinless
   chicken breasts,
   chopped into bite size
   chunks

4 cups fresh broccoli florets

1½ cups of your favorite
   shredded cheese

1. Preheat oven to 400°F; using extra-virgin olive oil, grease a 9x13-inch baking dish.

2. Add cauliflower, almond meal, your favorite seasonings, chicken broth, and milk to the dish and whisk together.

3. Add the chicken and broccoli, stirring to distribute into an even layer.

4. Cover and bake for 20 minutes.

5. Add the cheese to the casserole and stir well to combine; return to the oven for 20 minutes, uncovered.

6. Remove and stir stir once again, and cook for a final 20 minutes until chicken is cooked through (total baking time is 1 hour).

Batch and batch-base cooking can help save hours in the kitchen, and also ensure that you stick to your keto plan by being prepared. As you know, grain products such as bread, pasta, and pizza are not keto-approved, but if you're missing those we have you covered. In the next chapter, we will be introducing you to what is commonly known as a "game changer" in the keto community. Stay tuned!

Chapter 13

Your Keto Solution to Bread, Pizza Dough, Pancakes, and Waffles

If you're like millions of others, not having bread could cause you to completely derail from your *Super Simple Keto* plan. We have some delicious solutions for you and keto dieters swear by them! In this chapter you'll learn about keto-approved bread, pizza dough, pancakes, and waffles—a.k.a. "chaffles." These "bread" products are allowed on the *Super Simple Keto* plan because they are uniquely crafted to have the taste and texture of their wheat-based counterparts, but are made with keto-approved ingredients such as almond flour, coconut flour, cream cheese, and eggs. You will find a running theme of these ingredients throughout this chapter; however, there are different processes to achieve each outcome.

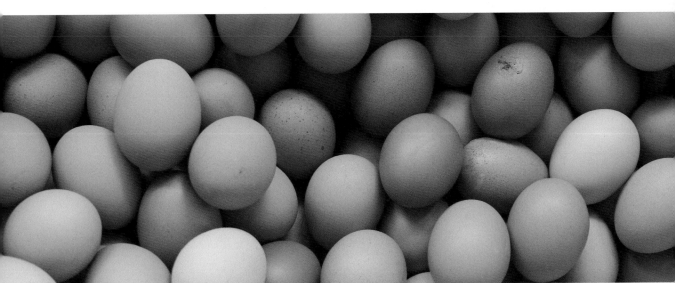

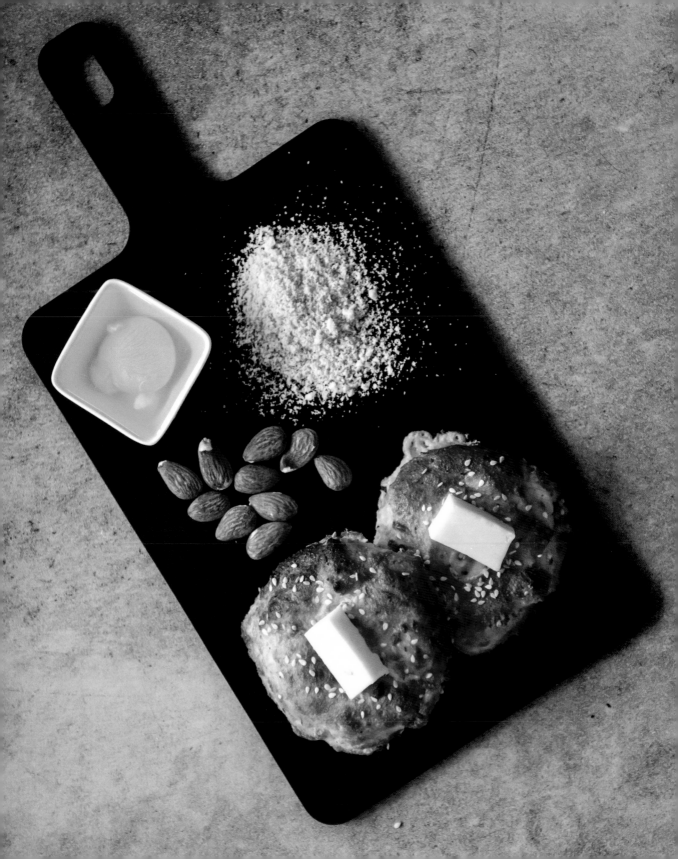

Keto Bread

If you hear the term "fathead" bread, it refers to lower-carbohydrate and higher fat breads which incorporates nut- and coconut-based flours as opposed to wheat flours. The term "fathead" comes from a 2009 documentary where high levels of fat and low levels of carbohydrates were consumed for the leading subject to lose weight. During the film, various doctors and dietitians interviewed stated that based on the latest research in cardiovascular health, it is actually inflammation (as opposed to a diet high in saturated fat) that causes heart disease and heart attacks; some of them stated that the inflammation is caused by a high-sugar, high-carbohydrate diet. This "fathead" bread dough is perfect for keto sandwiches, and can be made ahead of time and stored in the refrigerator before baking.

Makes 4 Sandwich Rolls

¾ cup shredded mozzarella cheese
2 ounces cream cheese
1 egg
⅓ cup almond flour
2 teaspoons baking powder
¼ teaspoon garlic powder
½ cup shredded cheddar cheese

1. Place the mozzarella and cream cheese in a microwave safe bowl. Microwave for 20 seconds at a time on high, until melted.

2. In a medium bowl, whisk the egg. Add the almond flour, baking powder, and garlic powder and combine.

3. Work the mozzarella mixture in with the almond flour mixture until sticky. Stir in the cheddar cheese.

4. Transfer the dough to a sheet of plastic wrap and fold plastic wrap over the dough. Gently work the dough into a ball. Refrigerate for 30 minutes.

5. Preheat the oven to 425°F and grease a baking sheet or line it with parchment paper.

6. Remove dough from refrigerator and unwrap. Cut dough into 4 equal pieces and roll each piece into a ball.

7. Cut each ball in half to form a top and bottom bun. Place the dough cut-sides down on the prepared baking sheet.

8. Bake until golden, around 10 to 12 minutes.

Keto Cloud Bread

Keto cloud bread is another version of a low-carbohydrate bread but it is far more light and airy. It doesn't have too much flavor on its own, so it's the perfect replacement for biscuits with butter or cheese, or for sandwich bread. Another bonus is you only need three ingredients as this bread does not call for any types of flour—not even nut- or coconut-based versions.

Makes 6 Pieces

Butter or ghee for greasing

3 large eggs, yolks and whites separated

⅛ teaspoon cream of tartar (optional)

3 ounces mascarpone or cream cheese, softened

⅛ teaspoon salt

1. Preheat the oven to 300°F. Line a baking sheet with parchment paper and grease lightly with butter or ghee.

2. In large bowl, beat the egg whites and cream of tartar with an electric mixer until you have stiff peaks.

3. In a different large bowl, use the electric mixer to beat the egg yolks, mascarpone or cream cheese, and salt until smooth.

4. Gradually (and carefully) fold the egg whites into the cheese mixture with a spatula. Try not to break down the air bubbles of the egg whites.

5. Scoop the mixture into six circular discs on the parchment paper and bake until golden, around 28 to 32 minutes.

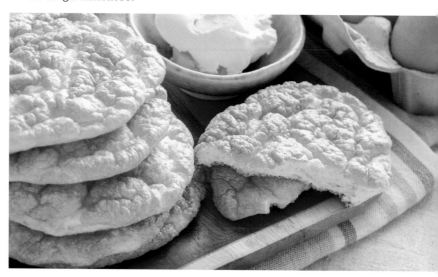

Keto Pancake

The keto pancake has almost the same ingredients as found in some of the waffles in the following "chaffle" section, however, if you do not have a waffle griddle, this recipe can be used for a pan. We don't necessarily condone the use of sugar-free syrups, but if you think they will work for you they can be added, or you can make a syrup-free pancake with heavy whipping cream and strawberries. You can also pair this pancake with a fried egg and mashed avocado for a savory breakfast dish.

Makes 1 Large Pancake

3 tablespoons almond flour
1 large egg
1 teaspoon baking powder
Splash of almond milk
Butter or ghee for cooking

1. Using a whisk, thoroughly combine all ingredients.

2. Heat a pan over medium-high heat and melt butter or ghee in the pan.

3. Pour the pancake mixture in the hot pan and wait until you see little holes in the batter as you would with regular pancake batter, around 2 minutes.

4. Flip the pancake over and cook for 1 minute, and serve.

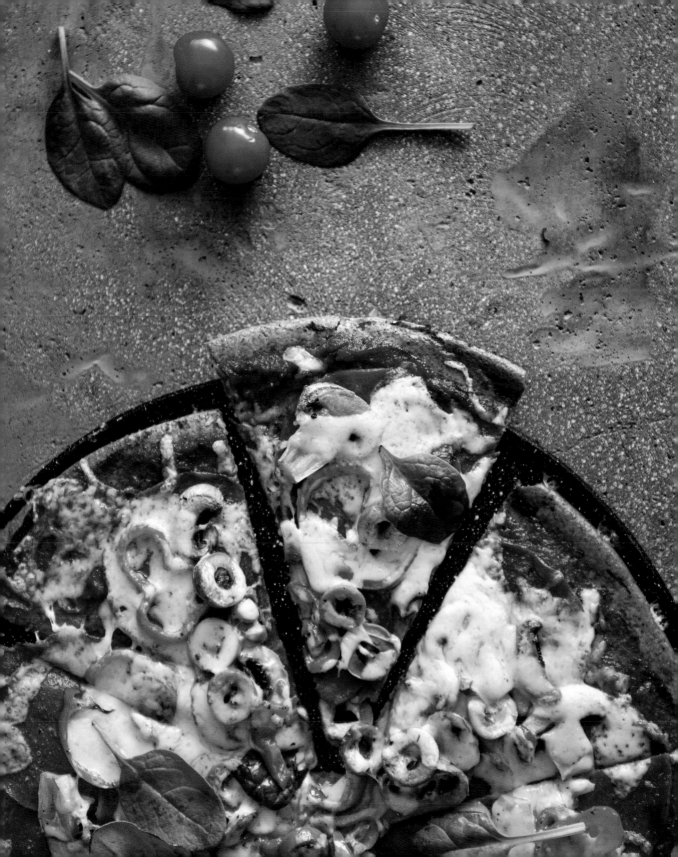

Keto Pizza Dough

Like with keto bread, you may hear keto pizza referred to as "fathead" pizza, and yes, it's the same thing! As with any pizza crust, the process is very important to get the dough just right. The biggest pointer is to keep kneading your dough until it is thoroughly combined and uniform. Also, if it's sticking to your hands, either chill the dough for 20 minutes to make it more manageable, and/or put some oil on your hands to make kneading easier. Feel free to use any keto-approved toppings on your pizza—cheese, sausage, pepperoni, bell peppers, and mushrooms are typical. For a low-sugar pizza sauce, refer to page 246!

Makes 1 Pizza Crust (8 Slices)

1½ cups shredded mozzarella

2 tablespoons cream cheese, cubed

2 large eggs, beaten

⅓ cup coconut flour

1. Preheat the oven to 425°F. Line a baking sheet or pizza pan with parchment paper.

2. Combine the shredded mozzarella and cubed cream cheese in a large microwave-safe bowl. Heat for 90 seconds on high, stirring halfway through. Stir again at the end until completely incorporated.

3. Stir in the beaten eggs and coconut flour. Knead with your hands until a dough forms. If the dough hardens before fully combined, microwave for 10 to 15 seconds to soften.

4. Spread the dough onto the lined baking pan to ¼- or ⅓-inch thickness, using your hands or a rolling pin over a piece of parchment paper to prevent the dough from sticking (the rolling pin and parchment paper method works best).

5. Use a toothpick or fork to poke lots of holes throughout the crust to prevent bubbling.

6. Spread low-sugar pizza sauce on top of the crust, followed by cheese, and toppings of choice.

7. Bake for 6 minutes. Poke more holes in any places where you see bubbles forming. Bake for 3 to 7 more minutes, until edges are golden brown.

The Chaffle

The chaffle is made with a mini waffle griddle so it looks just like a waffle and has a similar taste and texture. Many (but not all) chaffles are made using cheese, hence the name "chaffle" instead of waffle. The original chaffle appeared online not too long ago and it only has two ingredients: ½ cup cheese and 1 egg. Many love this version so we urge you to try it, but some argue this version is too "eggy" and doesn't have the bread texture they are looking for. This chapter provides several chaffle recipes that incorporate more ingredients to achieve the best bread-like texture.

Like we have mentioned previously, we don't endorse the use of artificial sweeteners or even natural zero-calorie sweeteners as it's imperative to get out of the habit of sweetening foods to kick the sugar habit. Due to this we don't use the chaffle for sweet purposes but rather for savory bread replacements—think of those delicious waffle sandwiches you see at specialty restaurants and amusement parks. There are several savory varieties of the chaffle taste-approved by thousands of keto dieters and some of the most common uses are included here.

Sandwich bread
Breakfast sandwiches
Grilled panini sandwich
Burger bun
Bagel
Pizza
Taco shells
Standard waffle

What You Need to Make Chaffles

The good news is you only need one piece of equipment: a mini waffle maker. Some make one mini waffle (or chaffle) at a time and some have two griddles or a double waffle maker which can come in handy. Either option will work, so it depends on how much you want to spend—the single waffle maker is around ten dollars and the double waffle maker is around twenty dollars at most major stores.

Popular Chaffle Recipes

The beauty of the chaffle is that the possibilities are endless. You can get creative and use your favorite ingredients to not only make the chaffle itself but also to form a new keto meal with it. Below you will find some of the most popular (and most delicious) chaffles made by many keto dieters. Simply combine all of the ingredients and use a nonstick cooking spray (we recommend keto-approved oil sprays as the best choices) to make one chaffle with your mini waffle maker.

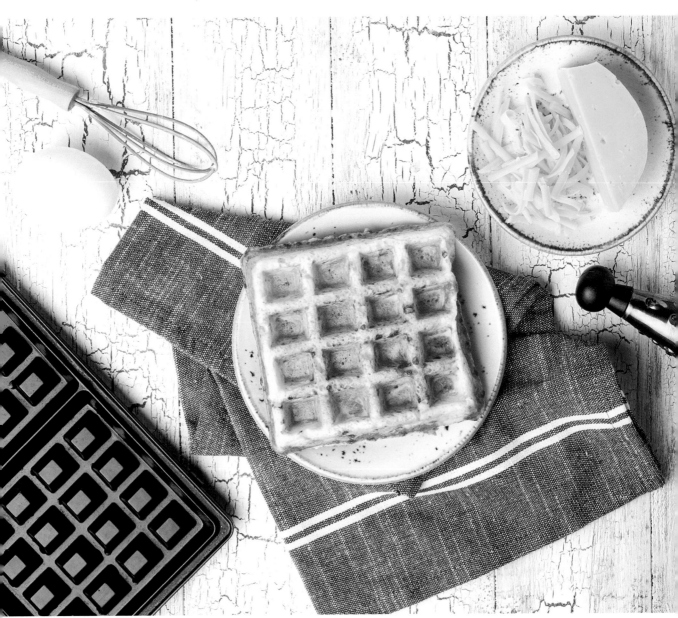

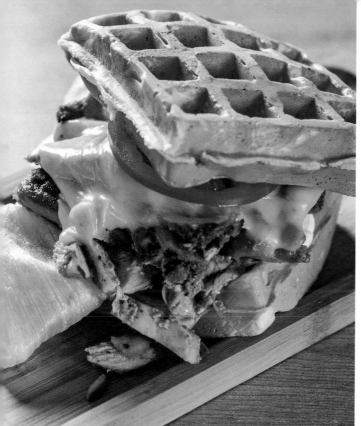

Wonder Bread Chaffle

So many keto dieters agree that this tastes just like white bread so you can use it as sandwich bread, a burger bun, or a grilled panini. Try it stuffed with pulled pork or beef, hamburger, or as a breakfast sandwich with egg, cheese, and bacon.

Ingredients:

3 tablespoons almond flour

¼ teaspoon baking powder

1 teaspoon water

1 egg

1 tablespoon mayonnaise

The Nut-Free Chaffle

This chaffle is the nut-free counterpart of the classic white bread chaffle found above. It will have the same taste but it's actually a little bit fluffier!

Ingredients:

1 tablespoon coconut flour

1 tablespoon water

1 tablespoon mayonnaise

⅛ teaspoon baking powder

1 egg

⅛ teaspoon salt

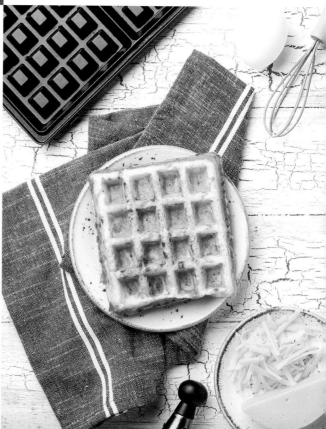

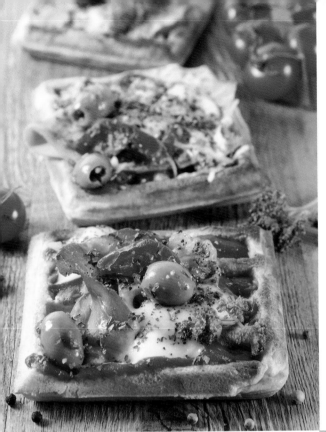

Pizza Chaffle

The pizza chaffle can be eaten on its own or you can top with more of your favorite pizza toppings such as extra cheese, tomatoes, olives, and prosciutto.

Ingredients:

1 egg
¼ cup Italian cheese blend
1 tablespoon Low-Sugar Pizza Sauce (page 246)
2 tablespoons pepperoni, diced

Lox Bagel Chaffle

If you love a bagel with cream cheese and lox, this is your chaffle! If you can't get your hands on the famous "Everything but the Bagel" seasoning, simply replace with a few dashes of sesame seeds, garlic powder, dried minced onion, and salt to taste. After making your chaffles, simply top with cream cheese and smoked salmon—other optional additions are sliced cucumber and/or radish.

Ingredients:

1 egg
¼ cup mozzarella cheese
1 tablespoon cream cheese
2 tablespoons almond flour
¼ teaspoon baking powder
Everything but the Bagel seasoning, to taste

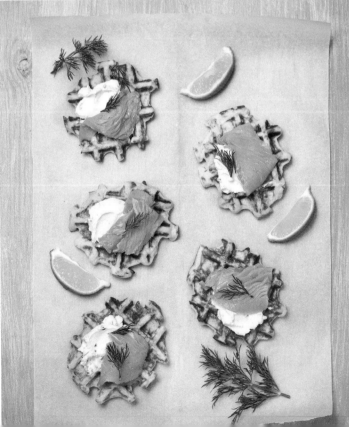

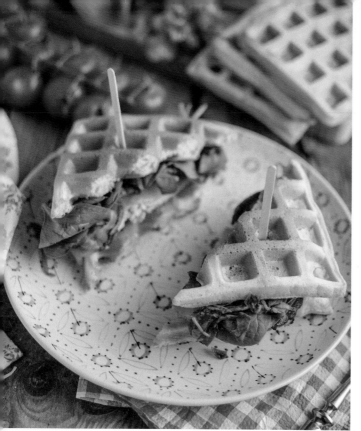

Stuffing Chaffle

If you like leftover holiday turkey sandwiches, you'll love the stuffing chaffle. Many elements of classic turkey stuffing are in this chaffle so this is the perfect "bread" for a turkey sandwich.

Ingredients:

3 tablespoons almond flour

¼ teaspoon baking powder

1 teaspoon water

1 egg

1 tablespoon mayonnaise

1 diced celery stalk + 1 tablespoon diced onion, sautéed

Poultry seasoning, sage, and thyme, to taste

Cheddar Chaffle

This chaffle has cheesy flavor so it is great for any sandwich where cheese may make a nice addition. Chicken salad and tuna salad sandwiches, BLTs, or standard ham and tomato sandwiches are popular ways to use this chaffle.

Ingredients:

1 egg

½ cup shredded cheddar cheese

1 teaspoon garlic salt

2 tablespoons almond flour

½ teaspoon baking powder

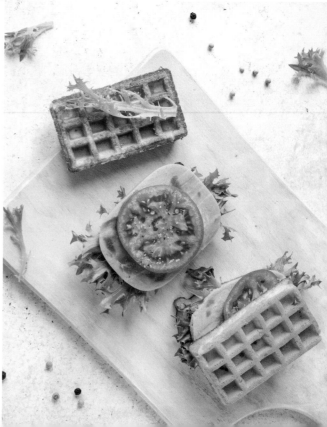

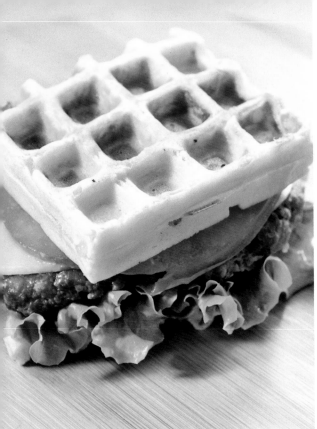

Mozzarella Chaffle

This chaffle is the mozzarella version of the cheddar chaffle and can be used in the same manner. It goes well with sandwiches and burgers, especially when mozzarella cheese is one of the additions.

Ingredients:

1 egg

½ cup shredded mozzarella cheese

1 teaspoon garlic salt

2 tablespoons almond flour

½ teaspoon baking powder

Standard Breakfast Chaffle

This is the recipe one would use if sugar-free sweetener and butter were added to make a breakfast chaffle. It's also a great pairing with eggs and mashed avocado as the chaffle acts as a bread component for the dish.

Ingredients:

2 eggs

2 tablespoons cream cheese

2 tablespoons almond flour

1 tablespoon coconut oil or melted butter

½ teaspoon baking powder

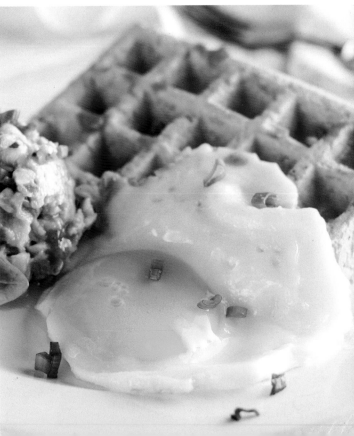

Batch Cooking the Chaffle

In the previous chapter about batch cooking, you learned how to make several meals in one cooking session that can be stored in the refrigerator or freezer. You can also implement this strategy with the chaffle as they keep well, and can simply be reheated by using your toaster. They may not be quite as crispy as the freshly made chaffles, but they come out pretty close!

We hope this chapter provided some variety in your nutrition plan with a keto-approved food that can double as bread, burger buns, bagels, and more. If you're like thousands of other keto dieters and love the chaffle, you can use it as a staple food and construct your meal plan around it. The recipes found in this chapter can be used for many simple ideas, and the possibilities are endless so feel free to use your favorite (low-carb and low-sugar) ingredients to make your favorite chaffle.

Chapter 14

Restaurant Keto

If you have absolutely no time for food prepping, or you just have zero interest or motivation to pack food for work, you can certainly eat in restaurants, order takeout, or even have the occasional fast food. In today's society, it's common to grab food (even every day!) during your lunch hour in a restaurant or at a takeout establishment. This is reality for many of us, so we want to provide a strategy for keto weight loss even if you're a frequent restaurant goer. Let's face it, life happens (and so do work luncheons, birthdays, and other social gatherings), and we want you to have options so you can live your life accordingly. Many think they have to give up their social lives or drastically rearrange their eating schedule at the office to adhere to the keto lifestyle, and that can lead to procrastination for even starting a nutrition plan due to strict limitations. Yes, you can still go to restaurants and enjoy wonderful company (and maybe even a glass of wine or two).

Fast food is permitted but we advise you to limit it to the odd occasion because we want you to achieve wellness in addition to weight loss. We have heard countless stories of keto dieters sticking to the proper macronutrients of fats, carbohydrates, and proteins by frequenting the fast-food drive through and ordering a bun-less double (or triple) cheeseburger with mayonnaise, along with a diet soda. It's an easy habit to get into since it's convenient, relatively cheap, and pretty tasty! Especially if you're new to keto and learning the ropes, we want to set the healthiest foundation possible and instruct readers how to get the best nutrition from this type of food plan since choosing detrimental foods (even while hitting your macronutrient requirements) can lead to unfavorable outcomes. Many people have reported adverse events such as drastically increased bad cholesterol, sodium, and even hospitalization when following a "dirty keto" nutrition plan which consists of a large percentage of fast food, deli meats, inferior oils, and processed foods. If you're in a true bind, then having one fast food meal per week (maximum) should not sabotage your health and wellness goals.

Dining establishments that are super simple and can be frequented often include:

- National chain dine-in restaurants.
- Smaller boutique dine-in restaurants.
- Takeout restaurants that offer salads, sandwiches (lettuce-wrapped), and platters with choices of unprocessed meats and vegetables.
- Coffee shops.

You'll want to limit regular use of:

- Standard fast-food establishments.
- Almost anything with a drive through.
- Pizza parlors.
- Takeout places that only offer processed deli meats.

It's convenient to look online at restaurant menus before choosing where to grab your meal as some have far more keto-approved options than others. If you end up somewhere without looking at food options first, not to worry—you can get a keto meal almost anywhere nowadays! Of course, you may have to modify your order, but making simple substitutions will turn a high-glycemic meal into a keto-friendly one quite easily. Below are thirteen common restaurant scenarios which include high-carbohydrate and high-sugar foods, as well as keto-friendly replacement options.

Scenario One:
You're at a typical café and the server arrives with a basket of bread and butter.

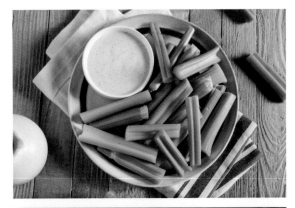

Solution 1: Before the bread even touches the table, just say "no thanks!"—you'll be eating a full meal soon anyway.

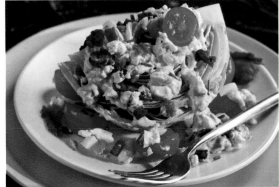

Solution 2: Replace with green veggies and a high-fat dip.

Solution 3: Replace with a small starter salad with a cream-based dressing.

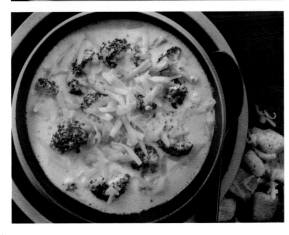

Solution 4: Replace with a low-carbohydrate, cheese- or cream-based soup.

Scenario Two:

You're at a more casual takeout place with sandwiches, salads, and burgers.

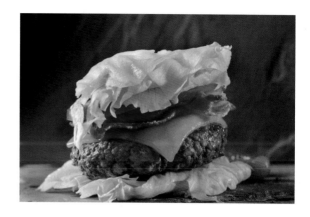

Solution 1: Just get it lettuce wrapped—most restaurants will oblige. Sorry, no fries, but a side of green vegetables will do!

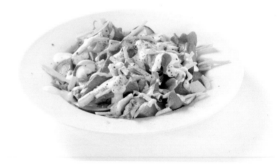

Solution 2: Not only will most takeout establishments lettuce wrap burgers, you can get sandwiches lettuce-wrapped too, or you can even ask for a "sub in a tub" to have all of your favorite sandwich fillings in a bowl.

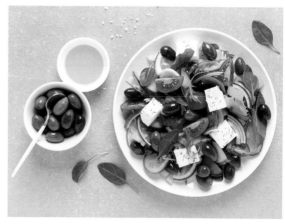

Solution 3: A hearty salad with fats that will keep you satiated—choose a dressing that is typically low in sugar such as oil and vinegar.

Scenario Three:
You're at an Italian eatery and everyone is getting pasta.

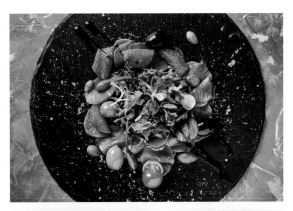

Solution 1: Beef carpaccio with additions such as arugula, cheese, olives, and tomatoes.

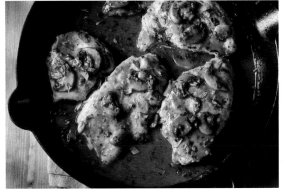

Solution 2: Any typical Italian protein dish such as chicken, meat, or fish, with no added pasta (feel free to sub in vegetables).

Solution 3: Caprese salad topped with olive oil.

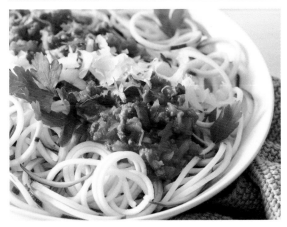

Solution 4: Not all, but many, Italian restaurants now offer zoodles (zucchini noodles) with meat sauce or meatballs. If this option isn't available, ask for meat sauce or meatballs with a side of green veggies or squash.

---

*Sorry, but no cauliflower crust pizza in restaurants is allowed—they are typically made with a mixture of wheat flour and cauli-flower.

Scenario Four:

You're at a typical chain restaurant with standard meals that contain a protein with side dishes of pasta, rice, and potatoes.

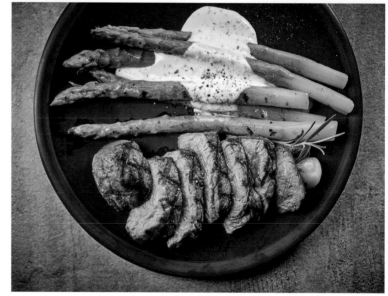

Solution 1: Ask your server to remove all high-carbohydrate side dishes and replace with low-carbohydrate produce.

Solution 2: Ask your server to remove all high-carbohydrate sides dishes and replace with one green vegetable with a cheese, cream, or butter-based sauce.

Scenario Five:
You're at happy hour with friends for drinks and small plates.

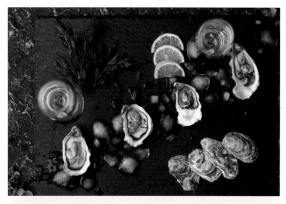

Solution 1: You celebrate your new keto lifestyle with brut sparkling wine and oysters.

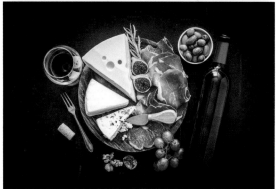

Solution 2: You relax with a glass of Cabernet Sauvignon and cheese board with nuts and olives.

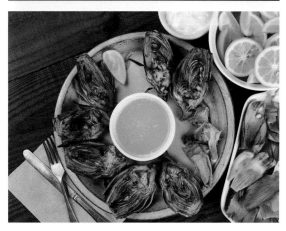

Solution 3: You pair a buttery Chardonnay with a steamed artichoke with mayo and butter for dipping.

Scenario Six:
You're grabbing Mexican food for Taco Tuesday.

Solution 1: Shrimp, steak, or chicken fajitas with guacamole, shredded cheese, and salsa—ask for lettuce cups or eat as a platter.

Solution 2: Chile verde platter of pork, green sauce, sour cream, and guacamole— skip the rice, beans, and tortillas!

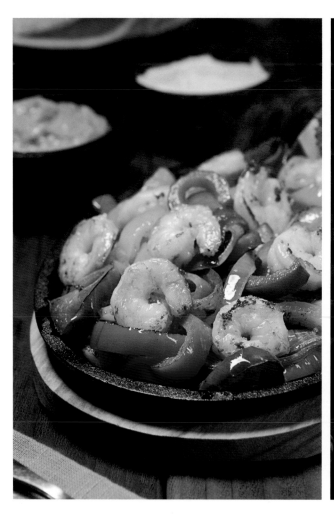

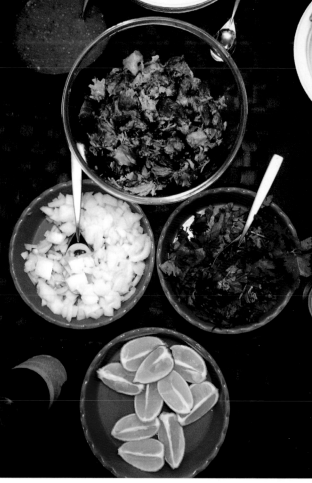

Scenario Seven:
You're out for Chinese or Vietnamese food, or for sushi.

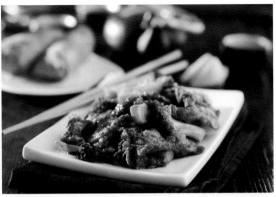

Solution 1: Beef and broccoli and egg drop soup instead of a noodle dish.

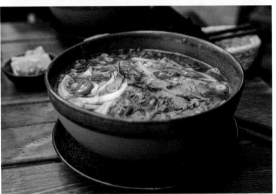

Solution 2: Vietnamese Pho (meat, noodle, herb, and vegetable soup)—ask for no noodles and extra veggies and herbs—this is a standard option on most menus!

Solution 3: At sushi, instead of a roll with rice, ask for it to be wrapped in cucumber—this, too, is a standard option on most menus!

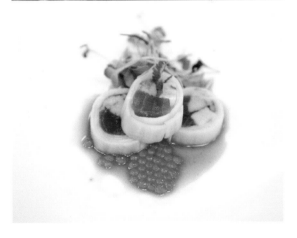

Scenario Eight:
You pop into Starbucks before work.

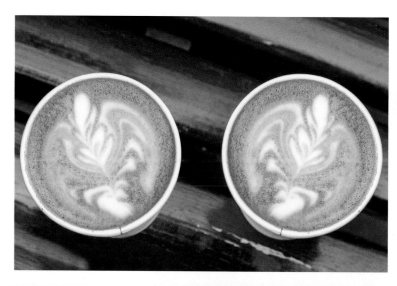

Solution 1: A grande coffee with heavy cream or almond milk, or a grande latte made with heavy cream instead of milk.

Solution 2: Egg bites (eggs with cheese and veggies, or eggs with cheese and bacon), string cheese, and mashed avocado. These items are offered ala carte and make an easy keto-approved breakfast on-the-go.

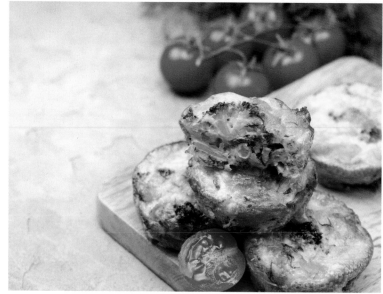

Scenario Nine:
You're out to breakfast or brunch with family and friends.

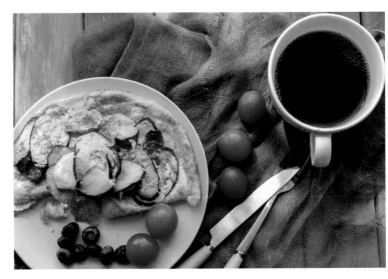

Solution 1: Omelet with vegetables, cheese, and sausage with small side of tomatoes and/or berries, and coffee.

Solution 2: Eggs Benedict with no bread base (most restaurants will make it this way); ask to add fresh produce such as asparagus, tomatoes, and mushrooms.

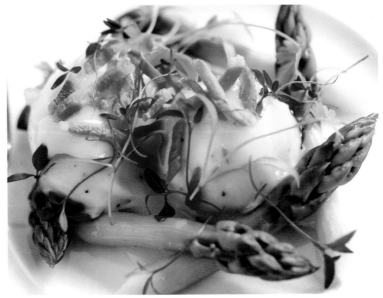

Scenario Ten:
You're at a sports bar watching Sunday football.

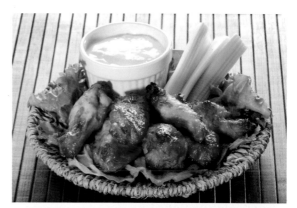

Solution 1: Wings, celery, and blue cheese.

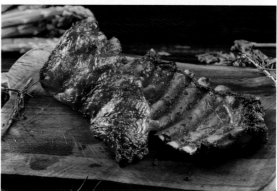

Solution 2: Baby back ribs (no sugary glaze) with green vegetables or a side salad.

Solution 3: Cobb salad with chicken or turkey, bacon, hard-boiled egg, tomatoes, avocado, and cheese.

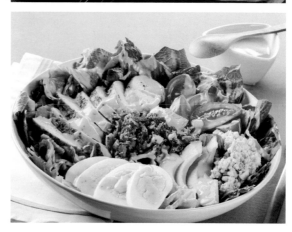

Scenario Eleven:
You're trying some Greek cuisine.

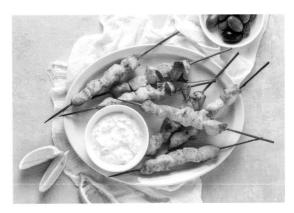

Solution 1: Chicken Souvlaki (kebabs) with cucumber yogurt dipping sauce and a side of olives.

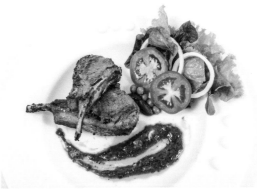

Solution 2: Lamb chops with side salad or green beans.

Solution 3: Gyro platter—skip the pita!

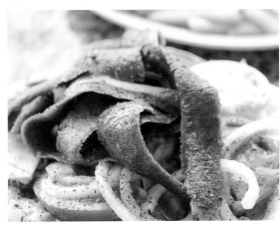

Scenario Twelve:

You're at a fine dining establishment to celebrate a special occasion.

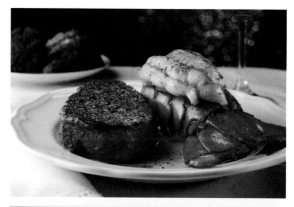

Solution 1: Steak and lobster with a green vegetable, and a glass of red wine.

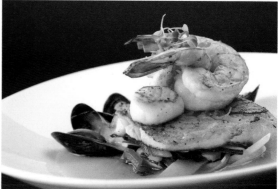

Solution 2: An eclectic seafood dish with fish, shellfish, and low-glycemic produce.

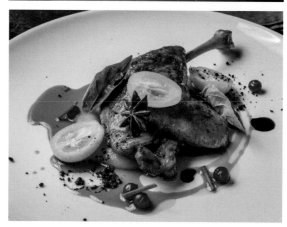

Solution 3: A fancy poultry dish such as duck confit with low-sugar fruits and greens.

Scenario Thirteen:
You pick a traditional steakhouse for some dinner.

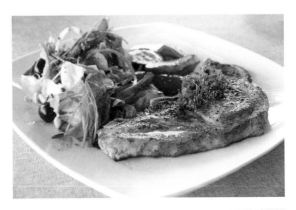

Solution 1: A juicy pork chop with vegetables and a side salad.

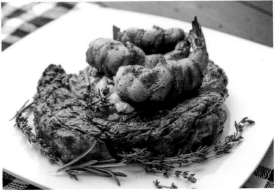

Solution 2: A ribeye with bacon-wrapped shrimp.

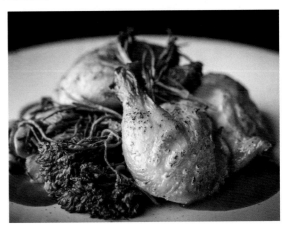

Solution 3: Roasted chicken with broccolini and mushrooms.

Contrary to popular belief, the keto nutrition plan can be achieved even if you frequent restaurants—you just have to be a little meticulous about your order! As with anything, once you establish a routine, ordering keto-friendly meals at any type of restaurant will become second nature. Of course, it's always best to prepare your own meals so you can choose the healthiest ingredients, but if that's just not realistic for your lifestyle, you can still get the weight loss results by following the simple guidelines found in this chapter.

Chapter 15

Super Simple Fast-Food Options

First and foremost, fast food is not the healthiest option and we are not, in any way, recommending the following establishments during your keto journey; however, if you're in a bind, this chapter details some of the best drive-through keto meal choices. We want to give you some on-the-go options if you find yourself in a pinch, but try not to take advantage of these keto fast-food meals more than once or twice per week as true health (not just weight loss) is our top priority for you. Just to have in your back pocket for emergencies, below you will find some of the most popular American fast food dining establishments, along with how to order keto-friendly meals at each one.

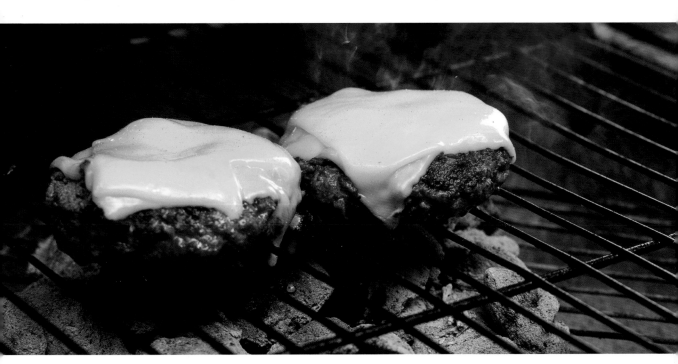

McDonald's

McDonald's has adjusted to the needs of its many keto customers. Essentially, you can order any burger or breakfast sandwich and simply say "no bun and no ketchup"—they will package your burger on a plate or bowl with meat, cheese, lettuce, a sprinkling of onions, and a slice or two of pickles. You can ask for mayo, ranch, and/or mustard on the side—sorry, but mainstream ketchup is a bit too high in sugar! The breakfast sandwiches will be served in the same way with egg, cheese, and sausage on plate. Keep in mind, you can use this McDonald's order strategy at most other burger-based fast food chains as they, too, are privy to the needs of keto dieters. There are at least twenty items to choose from at McDonald's but some of the most popular keto items can be ordered as follows:

- Any cheeseburger (single, double, triple) with no bun and no ketchup.
- Any breakfast sandwich with no muffin.
- Bacon Ranch Grilled Chicken Salad with no tomatoes and no dressing (sub ranch dipping sauce).
- Artisan grilled chicken sandwich with no bun. Sorry, but the nuggets and crispy chicken sandwich are off limits due to the chicken being encased in breading.

Subway

The term "sub in a tub" was coined at Jersey Mike's, but is often used at other fast food sandwich establishments. You can get your favorite sandwich fillings in a "tub" or bowl, without the bread. In addition to the sandwich bowls, Subway offers a variety of salads and breakfast items. Here's how to order some of their most popular keto items:

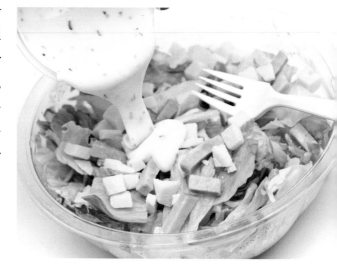

- 6-inch bacon, egg, and cheese sub with no bread.

- 6-inch tuna sub, plain with no bread.
- 6-inch cold cut combo sub, plain with no bread.
- 6-inch oven-roasted chicken, plain with no bread.
- Black forest ham salad.
- Chicken and bacon ranch salad.
- Spicy Italian salad.

Burger King

As with McDonald's, you can ask for any burger or breakfast sandwich with no bun and no sauce and it will be served on a platter or in a bowl. There are some other unique keto orders at Burger King below.

- Eggnormous Burrito in a bowl with no tortilla or hash browns; add a black coffee with cream on the side.
- You can replace French fry sides with a side salad, but remember to ask for no croutons.
- You can add ranch dipping or buffalo dipping sauce to any order.

Taco Bell

Just as you would order a burger with no bun, you can order tacos and burritos with no tortillas and Taco Bell will know what to do—you'll get a bowl or platter. To take it up even one more notch, there are keto-friendly power bowls that are loaded with additional ingredients such as guacamole and sour cream. Here are some of the most popular keto finds at Taco Bell.

- Steak or Chicken Burrito Supreme with no tortilla and no beans. You will get a bowl of protein, lettuce, diced tomatoes, diced onions, and a little bit of low-carbohydrate sauce.
- Chicken quesadilla melt with no tortilla. You will get a platter of melty cheese, chicken, and a little sauce to enjoy with a fork.
- The Grilled Chicken Power Bowl is packed with chicken, lettuce, guacamole, avocado ranch dressing, sour cream, and pico de gallo. Make sure to ask for no rice and beans, and feel free to add some hot sauce.

Wendy's

As with other popular fast-food chains, Wendy's is known for its burgers but they also have other keto-friendly items to choose from. Aside from the typical lettuce-wrapped burger order, here are some popular menu items. You can add the Caesar salad dressing, classic ranch dressing, or southwest ranch dressing to any salad or sandwich.

- Breakfast Baconator with no bun.
- Grilled chicken sandwich with no bun and no sauce.
- Southwest avocado grilled chicken salad.
- Parmesan grilled chicken Caesar salad.

Dunkin' Donuts

There is actually more to Dunkin' Donuts than just donuts, so if you're in a bind and need a quick breakfast, you can still pay them a visit (if the smell of the donuts won't derail your plan). Feel free to order any of their numerous hot and cold brews and unsweetened teas (just add cream). If you want to add a syrup to your drink, flavor shots are part of the secret menu and they are sugar-free (to learn more about sugar-free keto sweeteners, refer to chapter 11). You can order any of the following "Wake-Up Wraps" but just ask to hold the wrap.

- Sausage, egg, and cheese.
- Bacon, egg, and cheese.
- Ham, egg, and cheese.
- Turkey sausage, egg white, and cheese.
- Egg and cheese.

Chick-Fil-A

Just like ordering a burger with no bun, you'll do the same with the chicken sandwiches and breakfast sandwiches at Chick-Fil-A. There are some other notable items (besides the sandwiches) that are keto-friendly and here's how to order them.

- Hash brown scramble bowl with no hash browns and either grilled chicken or sausage.
- Grilled chicken nuggets with zesty buffalo sauce or garden and herb ranch sauce.
- Cobb salad with grilled chicken, topped with light Italian dressing or avocado lime ranch dressing.

Pizza Hut

Pizza parlors may be the most difficult to stay keto but there are a few options. If temptation is not a problem, you can order any pizza with lots of toppings and eat the toppings only. Sorry, but cauliflower crusts are not allowed in a pizza establishment because they are typically made with a percentage of alternative flour and a (usually) larger percentage of wheat flour. Here are a few non-pizza keto orders at Pizza Hut, and you will most likely find similar items at other pizza chains.

- Caesar salad.
- Chicken Caesar salad.
- Any order of wings with no breading and no glaze; add blue cheese or ranch for dipping.

Panda Express

Ordering keto at Panda Express can be tricky as many seemingly low-carb dishes are doused in sugary sauces. After meticulously going through their nutrition menu, you will find these to be the only suitable keto options, and of course all noodle and rice sides will need to be omitted.

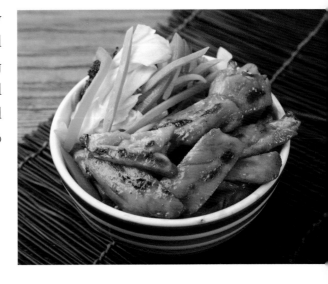

- Super greens entrée.
- Grilled teriyaki chicken.
- Grilled Asian chicken.
- Steamed ginger fish.

Sonic Drive-In

You'll use the same burger ordering techniques at Sonic since they have several burger and chicken sandwiches. There is one other unique keto option that you won't find at most other fast-food establishments and here's how you can order it.

- All-American hot dog with no bun, no relish, and no ketchup. The hot dog will be served with mustard and diced onions and if you need more than one, you'll still fall in line with your keto macros.

Chipotle Mexican Grill

Chipotle has really jumped on the keto wagon for their customers by adding a section of the menu called "Lifestyle Bowls." Here you will find several labeled keto bowls that have ingredients such as protein, cauliflower rice, avocado, and cheese, so you don't have to alter your order to make it keto. In addition, you will find other bowls labeled as "Paleo" and "Whole30" and those, too, are keto approved. Here are the most popular keto meals, and you can order them as is—simple as that.

- Keto salad bowl (served with greens, chicken, salsa, jack cheese, and avocado).
- Keto bowl (served with cilantro-lime cauliflower rice, chicken, salsa, jack cheese, and avocado).

Even if your favorite fast-food establishment was not found in this chapter, the techniques for ordering will remain the same for most other chains. Just remember the general rules of thumb—skip the buns, bread, tortillas, and fries, and beware of any high-sugar sauces. As a reminder, while you can still hit your keto macros with fast food, we suggest limiting these types of meals for when you're in a pinch for time so you achieve overall health and wellness, in addition to weight loss.

Chapter 16

The Plateau Solution: Keto with Intermittent Fasting

If you follow the proper caloric intake and macronutrients accurately, you should not hit a plateau, but that's not to say it can't happen. A plateau is when your weight loss results become stagnant for more than a few days. If you run into this issue, it's time to change it up and to reassess your nutrition plan.

If you do hit a plateau, before making any drastic changes, fully assess how you have been eating for the past week. If you have been truly sticking to your keto plan foods, the next step is to track every single calorie, gram of carbohydrate, gram of fat, gram of protein, and gram of sugar that goes into your body. You may find that maybe your nutrition plan hasn't been as targeted as you assumed. If it has been perfectly accurate in terms of carbohydrates, fats, and proteins, you may require fewer calories to achieve your ideal weight. If that's the case, try lowering your caloric intake by 300 to 500 calories per day and adjust your macronutrients (fat, carbs, protein) to fall into alignment with 70 to 80 percent fat, 10 to 20 percent protein, and 5 to 10 percent carbohydrates with your new/ lower calories as a guide.

If you're certain your nutrition plan doesn't need tweaking and you're just in a genuine plateau that your body won't snap out of, we would like you to try the solution found in this chapter, which is a very strict five-day keto plan paired with intermittent fasting. Intermittent fasting is a general term for various meal planning schedules that cycle between voluntary fasting and non-fasting over a reoccurring time period. Intermittent fasting is complimentary to the keto nutrition plan as ketones (the fuel we use to turn the gut into a fat burning machine) are increased during fasting. Also, when you are given a certain "feeding window," lower calorie consumption may naturally occur which can be an easy way to break a plateau. Studies and human trials do suggest that intermittent fasting may have beneficial effects on weight, body composition, cardiovascular bio-markers, and aging. At the cellular level, intermittent fasting may also increase resistance against oxidative stress, decrease inflammation, and promote longevity.[1]

There are several ways to employ intermittent fasting and some are much more doable for some than others. Below are five popular intermittent fasting schedules:

- **16/8 Method:** This involves fasting every day for sixteen hours, allowing food and beverage consumption (besides water) for only eight hours.
- **5/2 Method:** This involves eating a normal schedule of food for five days per week with no fasting on those days. The other two days per week will be restricted to 500 calories for women and 600 calories for men.
- **Eat Stop Eat:** This involves eating normally with no fasting for two days and then eating nothing for twenty-four hours and repeating that pattern.
- **Alternate Day Fasting:** This involves eating normally one day with no fasting and then eating only a few hundred calories the next day, repeating that pattern.
- **Spontaneous Meal Skipping:** This involves skipping at least one meal per day, not in any given pattern.

Given the *Super Simple Keto* plan, our preferred method of fasting is the 16/8 method because most of the fast takes place during sleeping hours, making it more realistic for people to achieve. We don't prefer any measures which include not eating for a full day or eating very little as that can lead to an unhealthy relationship with food, in addition to feeling so hungry that a binge could easily happen.

So you can really shake things up and get off this plateau you may be experiencing, we have put together a very strict five-day keto plan below that falls in the lines of the 16/8 intermittent fasting method, meaning you will have an eight-hour feeding window. Another approach is that you try the 16/8 method first along with the keto foods you have been consuming already. If that doesn't break your plateau, pair the 16/8 method with the following nutrition plan.

---

1   Stockman, Mary-Catherine, et al., "Intermittent Fasting: Is the Wait Worth the Weight?," NCBI, June 2018, https://www.ncbi .nlm.nih.gov/pmc/articles/PMC5959807/.

Your five-day sample intermittent fasting meal plan does not include calories or portion sizes—please adjust portions based on your calorie needs. Also, keep in mind that the following plan is a guide of suggestions; if you dislike a selection of food or have an allergy, please do not consume that particular food—just make a reasonable substitution. If there are particular meals or snacks you prefer, you can use them more than once and omit others.

16/8 Intermittent Fasting Keto Schedule
8-Hour Feeding Window: 10:00 a.m. to 6:00 p.m. (feel free to adjust as long as the window is eight hours, such as 11:00 a.m. to 7:00 p.m. or 9:00 a.m. to 5:00 p.m.)

Day 1

Before 10:00 a.m.: Any beverage with no calories such as water, plain tea, and black coffee.

10:00 a.m. Breakfast: Coffee with cream, butter, or ghee (optional), scrambled eggs topped with cheese and avocado slices.

12:00 p.m. Snack (optional): Celery and nut butter.

1:30 p.m. Lunch: Leafy green salad topped with 2 tablespoons olive oil, vinegar, canned tuna, diced red onion, and tomatoes.

3:00 p.m. Snack (optional): Olives.

6:00 p.m. Dinner: Chicken leg (with skin), zucchini cooked with olive oil, steamed cauliflower mashed with grated Parmesan cheese.

After Dinner: Any beverage with no calories such as water, plain tea, and black coffee.

Day 2

Before 10:00 a.m.: Any beverage with no calories such as water, plain tea, and black coffee.

10:00 a.m. Breakfast: Chia Pudding (page 175)

12:00 p.m. Snack (optional): Piece of cheese.

1:30 p.m. Lunch: Chicken tenderloins pan-fried in oil and seasonings with trio of dips: mashed avocado, mayonnaise, and Tzatziki (recipe on page 249).

3:00 p.m. Snack (optional): ¼ cup macadamia nuts or pecans.

6:00 p.m. Dinner: Steak topped with sautéed mushrooms and onions (use avocado oil or butter, white wine, garlic, and favorite seasonings to sauté), and side of roasted broccoli topped with oil, seasonings, and fresh lemon.

After Dinner: Any beverage with no calories such as water, plain tea, and black coffee.

Day 3

Before 10:00 a.m.: Any beverage with no calories such as water, plain tea, and black coffee.

10:00 a.m. Breakfast: Cottage cheese with berries and hemp seeds (optional). Coffee with cream, butter, or ghee (optional).

12:00 p.m. Snack (optional): ¼ cup Macadamia nuts or pecans.

1:30 p.m. Lunch: Egg salad in lettuce cups: Combine 2-3 diced hard-boiled eggs, diced celery, diced red onion, 2 tablespoons mayo, teaspoon of mustard, salt, pepper, and diced pickle (optional). Serve in lettuce cups or over a bed of greens.

3:00 p.m. Snack (optional): Salami slices with cream cheese and sliced pickles

6:00 p.m. Dinner: Salmon pan-cooked in butter and seasonings, paired with Brussels sprouts roasted in oil and seasonings.

After Dinner: Any beverage with no calories such as water, plain tea, and black coffee.

Day 4

Before 10:00 a.m.: Any beverage with no calories such as water, plain tea, and black coffee.

10:00 a.m. Breakfast: Smoked salmon rolled up with cream cheese and diced onion, paired with sliced tomatoes. Coffee with cream, butter, or ghee (optional).

12:00 p.m. Snack (optional): Celery sticks or endive leaves dipped in mashed avocado.

1:30 p.m. Lunch: Egg salad in lettuce cups: Combine 2-3 diced hard-boiled eggs, diced celery, diced red onion, 2 tablespoons mayo, teaspoon of mustard, salt, pepper, and diced pickle (optional). Serve in lettuce cups or over a bed of greens.

3:00 p.m. Snack (optional): Salami slices with cream cheese and sliced pickles

6:00 p.m. Dinner: Bun-less cheese burger topped with cheese, mayo, mustard, onion, and tomato with side of Parmesan roasted zucchini.

After Dinner: Any beverage with no calories such as water, plain tea, and black coffee.

Day 5

Before 10:00 a.m.: Any beverage with no calories such as water, plain tea, and black coffee.

10:00 a.m. Breakfast: Traditional bacon and eggs with side of berries. Coffee with cream, butter, or ghee (optional).

12:00 p.m. Snack (optional): Piece of cheese.

1:30 p.m. Lunch: Cobb salad with chicken or turkey, crumbled cheese, onion, tomato, avocado, and bacon (optional).

3:00 p.m. Snack (optional): 2-3 squares dark chocolate dipped in peanut butter.

6:00 p.m. Dinner: Grilled pork chops paired with sauerkraut.

After Dinner: Any beverage with no calories such as water, plain tea, and black coffee.

Remember to make a note of your plateaued weight before starting this regimented five-day intermittent fasting plan as you should see results in five days (or less). If this plan works for you, feel free to continue it as there is no danger in this type of intermittent fasting schedule. You can simply stick to your eight-hour feeding window while incorporating your preferred *Super Simple Keto* plan foods.

Chapter 17

The Keto Flu, Explained— and How to Combat It

Some people (certainly not all) may experience the "keto flu," which is a collection of mild symptoms that can be experienced when one transitions from a high-carbohydrate standard American diet to one that is far lower in carbohydrates. The keto flu is not, by any means, associated with actual influenza, but the name was merely coined by keto followers to describe the symptoms some experience when starting and adjusting to the diet. After years (or decades) of eating the same way, your body has grown to expect the same treatment and may even be sugar-addicted. When you adjust to a healthier lifestyle, cutting out these unnecessary sugars and extra carbs, the body can essentially rebel because it isn't being fed what it's used to.

Severely reducing your carbohydrate intake forces the body to burn ketones (instead of glucose) for energy. Ketones become the primary fuel source when following the ketogenic diet, and those ketones are byproducts of the fat breakdown. Usually, fat is used as a secondary fuel source when glucose is not readily available. This alternative of burning fat as opposed to sugar is called ketosis and can be achieved by adopting a very low-carbohydrate and low-sugar diet. This extreme decrease can come as a shock to the body, possibly causing withdrawal-like symptoms which present characteristics similar to ones experienced when weaning off an addictive substance. These keto flu symptoms, which may feel similar to the flu, can be a result of the body adapting to this process.

Keto Flu Symptoms

While many keto dieters never experience keto flu symptoms, if they do occur, signs of the keto flu typically start to arise within the first few days of drastically reducing carbohydrate intake. The switch to the ketogenic protocol is a major change and your body may need some time to adapt; however, the keto flu is no reason to be alarmed. Symptoms can range from mild to severe and may include one or more of the following:

- Nausea
- Constipation
- Diarrhea
- Headache
- Irritability
- Weakness
- Muscle cramps
- Dizziness
- Poor concentration
- Stomach pain
- Muscle soreness
- Difficulty sleeping
- Sugar cravings

The above-mentioned symptoms are commonly reported by those who have just begun the ketogenic nutrition plan. While the incidence of experiencing the keto flu varies from person to person, if you encounter any of the above symptoms, they typically subside after the first week of following the ketogenic nutrition plan. While these side effects may cause you to want to halt your keto endeavor, there are several ways to reduce them.

How to Get Rid of or Reduce Keto Flu Symptoms

If you experience the keto flu, don't give up yet, even if you feel like you want to! It can make you feel a bit off, but it will be short-lived and there are ways to alleviate any unsettling feelings. The following tactics are used by thousands of keto dieters to get through the ketosis transition period more easily.

Add Electrolytes

Electrolytes such as sodium, potassium, and magnesium may be depleted when one is in ketosis. When following the keto protocol, insulin (the hormone that assists with absorbing glucose from the bloodstream) decreases. The decrease in insulin levels causes excess sodium to be released from the body. Replacing dietary electrolytes has been shown to reduce keto-flu symptoms in many keto followers, so salting food may help with easing the keto flu.

Another electrolyte which can be lacking due to the keto nutrition plan is potassium since it is found in keto-restricted foods such as fruits, beans, and starchy vegetables and tubers. Consuming adequate amounts of potassium is another tactic to help adapt to the first week or two of consuming less carbohydrates. The keto-friendly avocado actually has more potassium than a banana so that is an ideal choice. Other keto-approved foods which are good sources of the electrolyte include those listed.

Another electrolyte to supplement to help reduce keto-flu symptoms is magnesium. Magnesium may help to alleviate sleep issues and headaches, as well as to reduce muscle cramps. Keto-approved foods which are good sources of this electrolyte include those listed.

Drink Lots of Water

No matter which nutrition plan one follows, staying hydrated with water is necessary for optimal health and wellness. Water also helps to reduce keto-flu symptoms as the keto diet can cause water storage depletion which can increase the risk of dehydration. Dehydration can be an added factor during ketosis because glycogen (stored

Potassium-Rich Keto Foods

Almonds
Brazil nuts
Cod
Cooked broccoli
Cooked spinach
Cucumber
Dried coconut
Flax seeds
Halibut
Hemp seeds
Leafy greens
Mushrooms
Pine nuts
Pistachios
Pumpkin seeds
Rockfish
Sunflower seeds
Trout
Tuna
Zucchini

Magnesium-Rich Keto Foods

Almonds
Avocado
Cashews
Chicken breast
Cooked spinach
Dark chocolate
Ground beef
Halibut
Peanut butter
Plain yogurt
Pumpkin seeds
Salmon

carbohydrates) is bound to water in the body. When glycogen levels drop by way of a reduction in dietary carbohydrates, water is excreted from the body. Replacing fluids (water is always your best bet!) may help with easing keto-flu symptoms such as muscle cramping and fatigue, and it will aid in overall wellness.

Take an Exercise Break and Get Rest

You can most certainly exercise on the keto diet but you may want to give yourself a little break if you experience keto flu symptoms. Your body is adapting to new fuel sources so during this time of transition, you should avoid activities like running, weightlifting, or any other high-intensity training. If you are not experiencing any keto flu symptoms, you can proceed with your normal exercise routine. If you are affected by the keto flu, a nice walk or leisurely bike ride may help improve symptoms.

Along with avoiding strenuous activity, make sure you are getting adequate amounts of sleep. Fatigue and irritability are common keto flu symptoms so getting your eight hours of sleep every night can help combat this. In general, lack of sleep can cause an increase in the stress hormone cortisol, and stress can intensify keto flu symptoms. Avoiding caffeine after 2:00 p.m. and ambient light from cell phones, computers, and televisions thirty minutes before bedtime can help with falling asleep more easily. In addition, waking up every morning at the same reasonable hour will assist with sleep regularity.

It's not common, but some keto dieters experience severe enough keto flu symptoms to cause them to stop keto altogether. If this happens to you, you may need to give your body more time to adapt by gradually easing into keto, and this means eliminating carbohydrates at a slower rate, rather than all at once. To learn how to slowly cut back on carbohydrates, while adding more fat and protein, refer back to chapter 8!

Chapter 18

The Super Simple "Keto Select" Meal Planning System

The Keto Select meal planning system is your simplistic guide to daily food recommendations that can be used when you need quick and easy ideas for breakfast, lunch, dinner, and snacks. You will be given different categories to select from which will lead to the proper keto macros on your plate. You may be wondering, *do I use the Keto Select meal planning system or the recipes found in coming chapters?* The meal planning system found in this chapter is a road map of basic food choices to follow and it's specifically designed for those who don't have time for recipes. If you find yourself on a lazy Sunday where

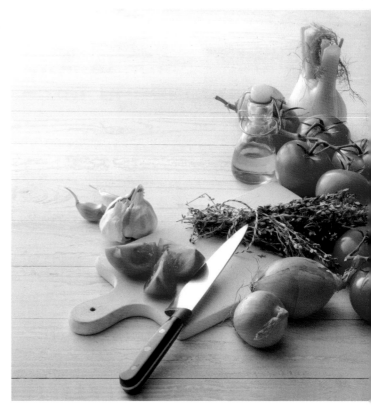

you do have some time to experiment, feel free to try the more complex breakfast, lunch, and dinner recipes found in the following recipe chapters.

Unlike the typical, rigid meal plan, the Keto Select meal planning system gives you several options for breakfast, lunch, dinner, and snacks—it's a "choose your own adventure" of sorts. At the beginning of each section (breakfast, lunch, dinner, beverages, snacks), you will be given a set of directions which will explain possible food options for that particular meal or snack. This will allow for some flexibility with regard to your taste buds, how hungry you are, caloric needs, and what you have in the pantry or refrigerator. The pick-four planning system is based on simplicity, convenience, and foods that are sound with regard to overall health, as well as weight loss. If you are feeling more adventurous, feel free to substitute any meal with one of the delicious recipes found in chapters 21, 22, and 23. Or you can even create your own unique daily food plans using the breakfast, lunch, and dinner recipes found in those chapters as all meals exhibited provide dense nutrition, while following the guidelines of the keto nutrition plan.

The items listed in the meal planning system are easily found in most grocery stores and the majority of the instructions (we won't even call them recipes) are easy, not calling for too many ingredients or too much preparation. We do not list every single keto-approved food in the meal planning system, so if you are wondering about appropriate substitutions, refer back to chapter 2 to make sure your food is allowed on your *Super Simple Keto* plan. If you're unsure of the appropriate serving size, the nutrition label of a particular food will list how much of the item should be consumed for one serving or you can refer the serving size chart found in chapter 4.

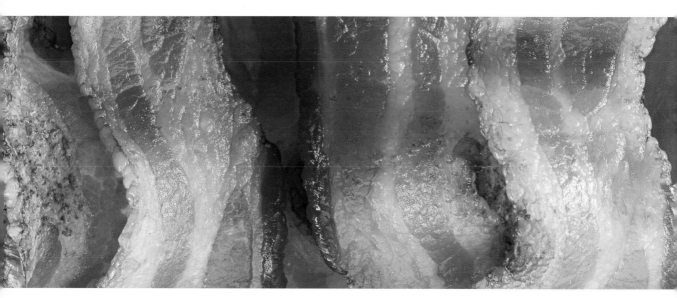

Food	Calories	Visual Cue
Vegetables		
1 cup green vegetables	25 calories	1 baseball
2 cups leafy greens (raw)	25 calories	2 baseballs
Low-Sugar Fruits		
½ cup berries	45 calories	1 tennis ball
½ cup sliced tomato	15 calories	1 tennis ball
½ cup sliced bell pepper	15 calories	1 tennis ball
Fats		
½ cup sliced avocado	115 calories	1 tennis ball
1 tablespoon oil	120 calories	3 dice
1 tablespoon butter	100 calories	3 dice
1 tablespoon ghee	135 calories	3 dice
1 tablespoon mayonnaise	103 calories	3 dice
6 ounces salmon	300 calories	2 decks of cards
1 ounce nuts	160–205 calories	2 golf balls
2 tablespoons nut/seed butter	95–175 calories	1 golf ball
1 cup full-fat yogurt	150 calories	1 baseball
1 cup full-fat cottage cheese	200 calories	1 baseball
1 ounce olives	60 calories	10 whole olives
Proteins		
6 ounces chicken/turkey	200–275 calories	2 decks of cards
6 ounces steak	320 calories	2 decks of cards
6 ounces fish	150–310 calories	2 decks of cards
6 ounces shellfish	130–170 calories	2 hands full
6 ounces ground beef	360 calories	2 decks of cards

Fatty Protein

1 to 3 Eggs Your Way: Choose your favorite preparation style—boiled, poached, scrambled, over-easy, or sunny side up.

1 or 2 Eggs Your Way with Smoked Salmon, Bacon, or Sausage: Choose your favorite egg preparation style and pair with 2 to 3 ounces of smoked salmon, 2 to 3 slices of uncured, nitrate-free bacon, or 2 to 3 pieces of breakfast sausage.

Smoked Salmon: 3 to 4 ounces.

Herring: 3 to 4 ounces.

Bacon: 2 to 3 pieces.

Breakfast Sausage: 2 to 4 ounces.

Steak: 4 to 8 ounces.

Cheese: 1 to 2 ounces.

Full-Fat Cottage Cheese: ½ cup to 1 cup.

Plain Full-Fat Greek Yogurt: ½ cup to ⅔ cup.

Plain Full-Fat Kefir: ½ cup to ⅔ cup.

Plain Full-Fat Coconut Yogurt: ½ cup to ⅔ cup.

Unsweetened Full-Fat Coconut Milk: ½ cup to ⅔ cup.

Plain Full-Fat Almond Yogurt: ½ cup to ⅔ cup.

Additional Fat

Avocado: ½, sliced or mashed.

Olives: ¼ cup.

Cheese: 1 slice of your favorite cheese or ¼ cup of your favorite shredded cheese, or 2 tablespoons cream cheese.

Nuts: 1 ounce almonds, pecans, pistachios, pine nuts, macadamia nuts, Brazil nuts, walnuts, or similar.

Seeds: 1 tablespoon chia seeds, flax seeds, hemp seeds, or sesame seeds.

Oils: 1 tablespoon healthy oil for sautéing.

Dairy: 1 to 2 tablespoons heavy cream, butter, or ghee.

Non-dairy: 1 to 2 tablespoons coconut milk or cream.

Nut/seed butters: 1 tablespoon nut or seed butter such as peanut butter, almond butter, cashew butter, Macadamia butter, or sesame butter.

Mayonnaise: 1 tablespoon avocado oil mayo or regular mayo.

Dressings & Sauces: 1 or 2 tablespoons of any high-fat, low-carbohydrate and low-sugar dressing or sauce.

Low-Glycemic Produce

Strawberries: 4 to 5 medium.

Blueberries: ½ cup.

Raspberries: ½ cup.

Blackberries: ½ cup.

Mixed berries: ½ cup.

Tomato: ½ cup, sliced.

Avocado: ½ , sliced or mashed.

Bell pepper: ½ cup, sliced or diced.

Mushrooms: ½ cup, sliced or diced.

Onions: ¼ cup, sliced or diced.

Spinach: 1 cup raw or ½ cup cooked.

Kale: 1 cup raw or ½ cup cooked.

Asparagus: 2 to 3 spears.

Broccoli: ½ cup to 1 cup, cooked.

Leafy greens: 1 to 2 cups.

Omelet Produce Mix (onions, bell pepper, mushrooms): ½ cup.

Example Breakfast Meals
Using the Keto Select Guidelines

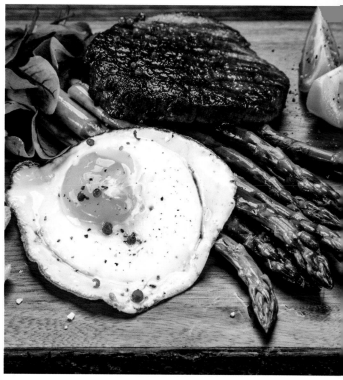

Keto Select Formula Sample 1:

Steak (fatty protein) +

Egg (fatty protein) +

Cooking oil (additional fat) +

Asparagus (low-glycemic produce) +

Tomato (low-glycemic produce)

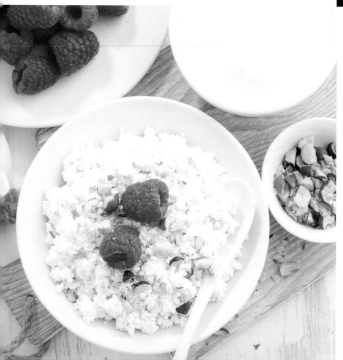

Keto Select Formula Sample 2:

Cottage cheese (fatty protein) +

Nuts (additional fat) +

Raspberries (low-glycemic produce)

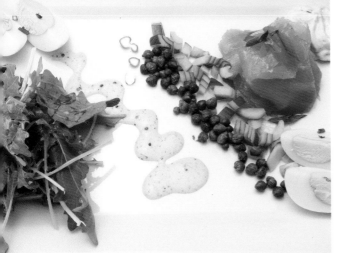

Keto Select Formula Sample 3:

Eggs (fatty protein) +

Salmon (fatty protein) +

Crème Fraîche (additional fat) +

Diced Onions (low-glycemic produce) +

Leafy Greens (low-glycemic produce)

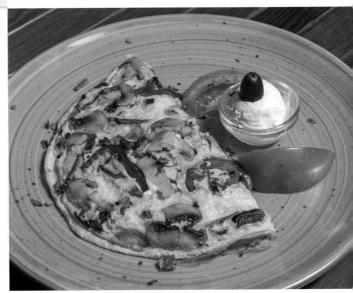

Keto Select Formula Sample 4:

Mushroom Omelet:

Eggs (fatty protein) +

Cheese (additional fat) +

Mushrooms (low-glycemic produce) +

Sour Cream (additional fat) +

Tomato (low-glycemic produce)

Keto Select Formula Sample 5:

Greek yogurt (fatty protein) +

Walnuts (additional fat) +

Strawberries (low-glycemic produce)

How to Meal Plan—Lunch and Dinner

Select one fatty protein or one lean protein. If you select a fatty protein, choose at least one or two additional fats. If you select a lean protein, choose at least two or three additional fats. Choose one or two selections from the low-glycemic produce category (optional).

Fatty Protein

Ground beef: 6 to 8 ounces.

Chicken or turkey with skin on: 6 to 8 ounces.

Salami: 2 to 4 ounces.

Ham: 2 to 4 ounces.

Pork sausage: 2 to 4 ounces.

Eggs: 2 to 3 whole eggs, prepared any style.

Cheese: 1 to 2 ounces.

Fresh or Canned salmon: 6 to 8 ounces.

Smoked salmon: 2 to 4 ounces.

Trout, Mackerel, or Catfish: 6 to 8 ounces.

Sardines: 4 to 8 ounces.

New York Strip, Rib-eye, T-bone, or Skirt Steak: 6 to 8 ounces.

Filet Mignon: 6 to 8 ounces.

Bone-in pork chops: 6 to 8 ounces.

Lamb chops or steaks: 6 to 8 ounces.

Lean Protein

Sirloin steak: 6 to 8 ounces.

Boneless pork chops: 6 to 8 ounces.

Boneless/skinless chicken or turkey: 6 to 8 ounces.

Deli turkey: 2 to 4 ounces.

Turkey sausage: 2 to 4 ounces.

Ground turkey or chicken: 6 to 8 ounces.

Canned chicken or tuna: 4 to 8 ounces.

Shrimp or Prawns: 4 to 8 ounces.

Crab, Clams, or Mussels: 4 to 6 ounces.

Snapper, Cod, Haddock, Sole, Halibut, or Swordfish: 6 to 8 ounces.

Additional Fat

Avocado: ½, sliced or mashed.

Olives: ¼ cup.

Cheese: 1 slice of your favorite cheese or ¼ cup of your favorite shredded cheese, or 2 tablespoons cream cheese.

Nuts: 1 ounce almonds, pecans, pistachios, pine nuts, macadamia nuts, Brazil nuts, walnuts or similar.

Seeds: 1 tablespoon chia seeds, flax seeds, hemp seeds, or sesame seeds.

Oils: 1 tablespoon healthy oil for sautéing.

Dairy: 1 tablespoon heavy cream, butter, or ghee.

Non-Dairy: 1 to 2 tablespoons coconut milk or cream.

Nut/seed butters: 1 tablespoon nut or seed butter such as peanut butter, almond butter, cashew butter, Macadamia butter, or sesame butter.

Bacon: 1 to 2 strips.

Mayonnaise: 1 tablespoon avocado oil mayo or regular mayo.

Dressings & Sauces: 1 or 2 tablespoons of any high-fat, low-carbohydrate and low-sugar dressing or sauce.

Low-Glycemic Produce

Zucchini: 1 cup, cooked.

Spaghetti Squash: 1 cup, cooked.

Fennel: ½ to 1 cup, cooked.

Tomato: ½ cup, sliced.

Avocado: ½, sliced or mashed.

Bell pepper: ½ cup, sliced or diced.

Mushrooms: ½ cup, sliced or diced.

Onions: ¼ cup, sliced or diced.

Hot peppers: ½ cup, sliced.

Pickles: ½ cup, sliced.

Spinach: 1 cup raw or ½ cup cooked.

Kale: 1 cup raw or ½ cup cooked.

Asparagus: 3 to 4 spears.

Green beans: 1 cup, cooked.

Broccoli: ½ to 1 cup cooked.

Brussels sprouts: ½ to 1 cup cooked.

Cucumber: ½ to 1 cup, sliced.

Leafy greens: 1 to 2 cups.

Cabbage: 1 to 2 cups.

Burger topper combo: 2 to 3 lettuce leaves, 1 large slice tomato, 1 thin slice onion.

Small mixed salad: 1 to 2 cups leafy greens, ⅓ cup diced tomato/onion, 1 half avocado, sliced.

Sandwich lettuce cup combo: 2–4 large lettuce leaf cups, ⅓ cup diced tomato/onion, ½ avocado, sliced.

Mixed produce: 1 to 2 cups any mixed low-glycemic produce.

Example Lunch and Dinner Meals Using the Keto Select Guidelines

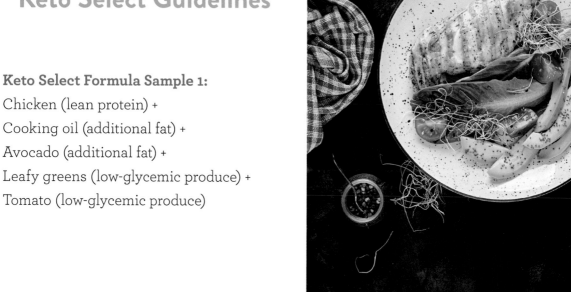

Keto Select Formula Sample 1:

Chicken (lean protein) +

Cooking oil (additional fat) +

Avocado (additional fat) +

Leafy greens (low-glycemic produce) +

Tomato (low-glycemic produce)

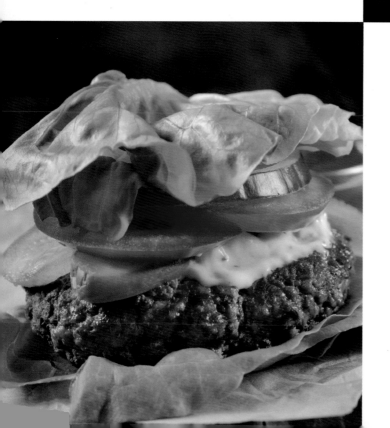

Keto Select Formula Sample 2:

Ground Beef (fatty protein) +

Mayonnaise (additional fat) +

Burger Topper Combo (low-glycemic produce) +

Pickles (low-glycemic produce)

Keto Select Formula Sample 3:

Eggs (fatty protein) +

Mayonnaise (additional fat) +

Leafy greens (low-glycemic produce)

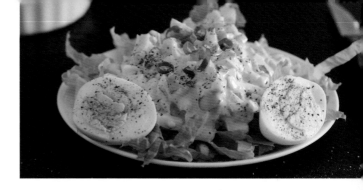

Keto Select Formula Sample 4:

Shrimp (lean protein) +

Avocado (additional fat) +

Pesto (additional fat) +

Parmesan cheese (additional fat) +

Spinach (low-glycemic produce) +

Zucchini noodles (low-glycemic
  produce)

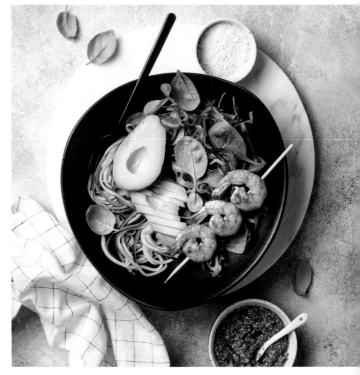

Keto Select Formula Sample 5:

Ground Chicken (lean protein) +

Cooking Oil (additional fat) +

Cheese (additional fat) +

Cucumber (low-glycemic produce) +

Burger Topper Combo (low-glycemic
  produce)

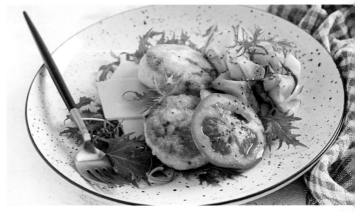

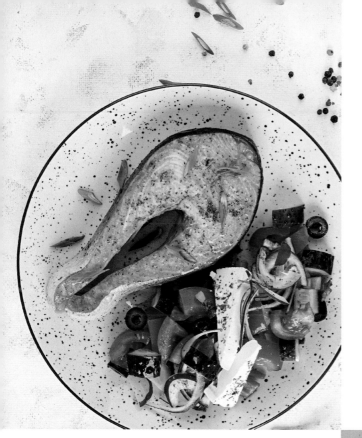

Keto Select Formula Sample 6:
Salmon (fatty protein) +
Feta cheese (additional fat) +
Olives (additional fat) +
Mixed produce (low-glycemic produce)

Keto Select Formula Sample 7:
Steak (fatty protein) +
Loaded cauliflower: cauliflower
   (low-glycemic produce) +
Cheese (additional fat) +
Bacon (additional fat) +
Asparagus (low-glycemic
   produce)

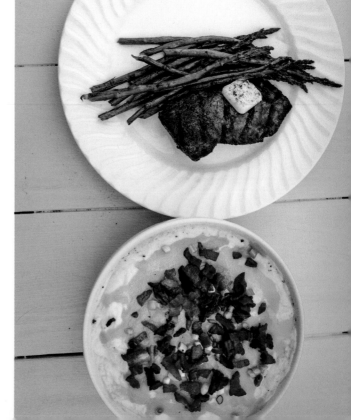

As a reminder, not all keto-approved foods are found in this chapter—please refer to chapter 4 if you're looking for additions or substitutions. The Keto Select Meal Planning System employs common, easy-to-find foods that most mainstream grocery stores carry. For a variety of unique breakfast, lunch, dinner, side dish, sauce, and dressing recipes, refer to chapters 21 through 24.

Chapter 19

Niche Keto Foods
to Know About

There are several foods in the ketogenic world that are quite unique and possibly even unheard of in some parts. If you haven't heard of many of the niche keto foods or are unsure of what they are used for, you are not alone. The purpose of this chapter is to outline and explain popular high-fat, low-carbohydrate, low-sugar items that may not be ones you, personally, have ever had in your grocery cart. The following list merely gives you more options that will help you achieve your keto plan macronutrient breakdown. If you are doing fine on your own with more mainstream foods, don't feel obligated to purchase or use any of the below foods. If you're looking for more options or you want to get more creative in the kitchen, you may find this chapter beneficial.

Coconut Oil

Extracted from the meat of mature coconuts, coconut oil is very popular in the keto community as its fat profile is different than most other cooking oils. Typically, fats in the diet come from long-chain triglycerides, however, the fats found in coconut oil are called medium-chain triglycerides (MCTs) as these fats are shorter, having between six and twelve carbons. There are four primary MCTs that are categorized, based on their carbon lengths—C6 (caproic acid) contains six carbons, C8 (caprylic acid) contains eight carbons, C10 (capric acid) contains ten carbons, and C12 (lauric acid) contains twelve carbons. Because of their chemical structure, MCTs go to the liver where they are used as a quick source of energy, and they can increase fat burning, as well as raise your HDL (good) cholesterol.[1] Coconut oil provides a mixture of all medium-chain triglycerides, and is most abundant in C12 (lauric acid). Once digested, lauric acid helps create mono-laurin which helps kill harmful bacteria, viruses, and fungi.[2] Coconut oil can be used for cooking at high heat, creamer for coffee, added nutrients in smoothies, and moisturizing the skin without added chemicals.

MCT Oil

The primary difference between coconut oil and MCT oil is that coconut oil is comprised of around 55 percent medium-chain triglycerides, whereas MCT oil is 100 percent medium-chain triglycerides. In addition, while C12 (lauric acid) is beneficial to fend off harmful bacteria, viruses, and fungi, it is the most prevalent MCT found in coconut oil. Since it is the longest MCT, it is the least efficient in terms of converting to ketones. For greater ketone conversion, MCT oil contains a much higher proportion of C8 (caprylic acid) and C10 (capric acid) which are known for brain health and curbing hunger. These specific MCTs will give you the benefits of a strict ketogenic nutrition plan, while being able to consume more carbohydrates. A 2015 meta-analysis found that MCTs helped to decrease weight, hip and waist circumference, visceral fat, and total body fat.[3] MCT oil has no taste or smell and can be taken on its own or added to coffee, smoothies, and salad dressings.

Keto Coffee

Keto coffee is a high-fat, high-calorie coffee that is typically made with brewed coffee, grass-fed butter or ghee, and MCT oil. It is suggested to use a blender to thoroughly

---

1   Chinwong, S., D. Chinwong, and A. Mangklabruks. "Daily Consumption of Virgin Coconut Oil Increases High-Density Lipoprotein Cholesterol Levels in Healthy Volunteers: A Randomized Crossover Trial." NCBI. December 14, 2017. Accessed May 19, 2019. https://www.ncbi.nlm.nih.gov/pmc/articles/PMC5745680/.

2   Kabara, J., D. Swieczkowski, A. Conley, and J. Truant. "Fatty Acids and Derivatives as Antimicrobial Agents." NCBI. July 1972. Accessed May 19, 2019. https://www.ncbi.nlm.nih.gov/pmc/articles/PMC444260/.

3   Mumme, K., and W. Stonehouse. "Effects of Medium-chain Triglycerides on Weight Loss and Body Composition: A Meta-analysis of Randomized Controlled Trials." NCBI. February 2015. Accessed May 19, 2019. https://www.ncbi.nlm.nih.gov/pubmed/25636220.

combine the ingredients for a smooth and frothy texture. Since bullet proof coffee does offer a substantial amount of fat and calories, some choose to use the coffee as a breakfast replacement. For a simple Keto Coffee recipe, see page 177.

Dark Chocolate

Dark chocolate is an acceptable keto dessert or snack as it is high in fat, while remaining low in sugar. Be sure to choose a minimum of 75 percent cocoa solids as the higher the cocoa content, the lower the sugar. One glass of red wine has 1 to 2 grams of sugar so the pairing of dark chocolate with your favorite Cabernet will make the perfect keto-friendly dessert.

Seaweed

Seaweed is a less commonly consumed vegetable, and it is one of the best vegan sources of Omega-3 fatty acids. Seaweed and other marine algae actually have even more concentrated vitamins and minerals compared to vegetables that are grown on land. An excellent source of vitamins K, B, zinc, iron, as well as antioxidants, seaweed can be eaten on its own, as a side dish, or in salads.

Hemp Seeds

Hemp seeds have a very mild nutty flavor and almost go unnoticed when added to dishes as they are so subtle, with a delicate (non-crunchy) texture. Three tablespoons of hemp seeds boast 15 grams of fat, many of which come from omega-3 fatty acids. They are also an excellent source of iron, thiamin, phosphorus, magnesium, and manganese. You can sprinkle hemp seeds on salads, yogurt, or in smoothies.

Ground Psyllium Husk Powder

Psyllium is a type of fiber that is formed from the husks of the *Plantago ovata* plant's seeds. A natural laxative, many studies show that taking this supplement is beneficial for digestion, as well as heart and pancreas health. The powder is gluten-free and low-carbohydrate and is used for keto baking. The psyllium husk acts like a binder and helps keto-friendly breads have the same type of texture and consistency as traditional baked goods. This ingredient is a staple in keto baking as it causes bread to hold more moisture and achieve a light, airy consistency.

Coconut Flour

Coconut flour is a naturally grain-free and gluten-free flour that is made from dried coconut meat—coconut milk production results in the byproduct of coconut flour. Rich in medium chain triglycerides, it can help to achieve and maintain ketosis, and also promotes good digestion, heart health, and stable blood sugar. High in protein and fiber, while remaining low in carbohydrates, coconut flour is popular in the keto and paleo communities for baking.

Shirataki Noodles

Shirataki are thin and translucent Japanese noodles made from glucomannan, a fiber that comes from the root of the konjac plant. Shirataki are comprised of 97 percent water and 3 percent glucomannan; many studies suggest that glucomannan is associated with weight loss, as well as body fat and cholesterol reduction.[4] Besides noodles made from squash and zucchini, these are the only true pasta-like noodles that are acceptable in the keto and paleo communities as they are low in calories and carbohydrates, while still high in fiber.

Nutritional Yeast

Nutritional yeast is a deactivated yeast with a cheesy flavor, found in flake or powder form. It is vegan-friendly and a substantial source of fiber, amino acids, and vitamin B12. Since it is very low in carbohydrates and sugar, it makes the perfect addition to the keto nutrition plan, especially if one is dairy-free. Sprinkle on salads and entrees for added

---

4   Kaats, G. R., D. Bagchi, and H. G. Preuss. "Konjac Glucomannan Dietary Supplementation Causes Significant Fat Loss in Compliant Overweight Adults." NCBI. October 22, 2015. Accessed May 20, 2019. https://www.ncbi.nlm.nih.gov/pubmed/26492494.

savory flavor, or made into a plant-based cheese sauce (see page 250), it makes a wonderful addition to many dishes.

Tahini

Tahini is a creamy nondairy butter that is made strictly from sesame seeds. In addition to being plant-based, tahini is high in healthy fats, moderate in protein and fiber, and low in carbohydrates. It's also packed with nutrients including copper, manganese, calcium, magnesium, iron, zinc, selenium, and thiamin. Tahini can be used in dips, sauces, smoothies, and salad dressing, or alone as a seed butter—refer to page 255 for our Creamy Tahini-Lemon Dressing.

Ghee

Ghee is clarified butter that is made by heating butter to separate the liquid and milk portions from the fat. The milk turns in to a solid, and the remaining oil is ghee. Since the milk separates from the oil, ghee is dairy-free and has a much higher smoke point than butter. Ghee can be melted over vegetables, used in Keto Coffee (see page 177), or used in place of oil or butter when cooking dishes such as stir fry or eggs.

Bone Broth

Bone broth is made by simmering the bones and connective tissues of beef, pork, lamb, turkey, chicken, bison, venison, or fish. It is more nutrient-dense than standard broth and stock due to its longer cooking time; however, the nutrient content is determined by the bones used in the broth. Animal bones are packed with calcium, magnesium, potassium, and phosphorus, whereas fish bones also contain iodine, which is important for metabolism and thyroid function. Connective tissues provide glucosamine and chondroitin which support joint health, and marrow supplies vitamin A, vitamin K2, zinc, iron, boron, manganese, and selenium, as well as omega-3 fatty acids. The above-mentioned components also contain the protein collagen, which turns into gelatin when cooked and produces numerous essential amino acids. As the ingredients simmer, the water absorbs the nutrients, so the vitamins and minerals can be consumed via drinking bone broth on its own or from being incorporated in soups, sauces, and gravies.

Avocado Oil Mayo

Regular mayonnaise can be used in your keto nutrition plan, but avocado oil mayo (or sometimes called "paleo mayo") has a healthier fat composition due to the fact that avocado oil is superior to the oils used in standard commercial mayonnaise. Avocado oil mayo is higher in monounsaturated fats and extremely low in sugar and carbohydrates—it can be pricey in some grocery stores so please refer to page 250 to learn how to make your own. Avocado oil mayo can be used in tuna salad, for dipping roasted vegetables such as artichokes, or as a creamy base for salad dressing.

We hope this chapter has been useful for you with regard to learning about foods that are often talked about in keto communities. Like we mentioned earlier, you don't need to incorporate these items in your nutrition plan; however, some can be very helpful for achieving your keto macronutrient combination. Not to mention, many find these additions to be unique and delicious, providing more variety in your grocery cart and meal plans.

Chapter 20

Unhealthy "Health Foods"

For decades, we have been told to eat particular foods in order to increase intake of certain vitamins, as well as to achieve specific health and wellness goals. Unfortunately, some of these foods that have been touted as superior sources of the nutrients we need are actually lower quality than what we have been led to believe by extensive marketing efforts. The unhealthy health foods listed below are either packed with sugar, high in carbohydrates, or have been laden with general blanket statements that have little to no credible statistics or research to back them up. Unfortunately, these detrimental foods are some of the primary culprits in the deteriorating health of the general population, and powerful marketing has resulted in voluminous consumption by the masses.

Flavored Yogurts

Some yogurts can be incorporated into your ketogenic plan but you must have a good look at the nutrition and ingredients label to ensure you're not packing in the same amount of sugar (or sometimes more) as you would with a bowl of ice cream. Flavored and low- or nonfat yogurts tend to be the biggest offenders with upwards of 47 grams of sugar per cup, which exceeds the limit of daily sugar intake for men and women in just one serving. It is best to choose full-fat, plain yogurt and be sure to check the label to make sure there is no added sugar by way of high-fructose corn syrup or other sweeteners.

Protein Bars

Just like yogurt, some protein bars are formulated to meet ketogenic standards, but the majority are not. Many contain as much as 30 grams of sugar per bar which is equivalent to eating a standard candy bar. If you do enjoy snacking on a protein bar, check the label for high fat content and extremely low sugar—typically, these keto-friendly protein bar ingredients include items such as coconut oil, almond butter, coco butter, medium-chain triglyceride (MCT) oil, and collagen.

Granola

Granola tends to be classified as a nutritious health food but most commercial brands include a variety of sweeteners in one brand. All three—cane sugar, brown rice syrup, and tapioca syrup—are found in popular commercial brands of granola. Unfortunately, it is commonplace to top flavored yogurt with these sweetened grain mixtures resulting in a small meal that contains as much as 63 grams of sugar. If you're a granola fan, there are many keto renditions that include ingredients such as nuts, seeds, coconut, coconut oil, and vanilla extract.

Kombucha

Kombucha is ancient, fermented tea and provides a host of benefits through its probiotic content, however, some brands have as much as 20 grams of sugar per serving, which is almost comparable to the sugar content of soda. If you're looking for the gut and microbiome benefits that kombucha can provide, choose unflavored selections which have less than 4 grams of sugar per serving.

Cereal Bars

Like cereal, cereal bars are touted as "heart healthy," yet are packed with added sugars and highly processed ingredients. The nutritional value of the processed ingredients is so low that most cereal bars are fortified with fake synthetic nutrients as the processing kills many of the naturally occurring vitamins and minerals.

Premade Soups

Soups are a wonderful part of the keto nutrition plan when using ingredients such as coconut milk, avocado, vegetables, and proteins, but if you're looking for a quick low-carbohydrate and low-sugar soup found in a can, you will really have to inspect the nutrition label. For example, one can of Campbell's classic tomato soup has 20 grams of sugar—the same as two glazed donuts! Not all canned soups are sugar culprits so with some label checking, you may be able to find some convenient pre-made options.

Vitamin Water

Vitamin water is marketed as healthy since it contains a variety of added synthetic nutrients (some of which can be hard to absorb). Another addition to these drinks is sugar—one bottle has as much as 32 grams which is comparable to the amount of sugar found in soda. It's best to stick to water or unsweetened sparkling water during your keto plan.

Canned Baked Beans

Beans and legumes aren't regularly consumed in the keto world; however, if you're on point with measuring your carbohydrate intake, you may be able to squeeze a small portion in. This doesn't mean canned baked beans though! Canned baked beans are known for their sweet and tangy flavor because only ½ cup packs 10 grams of sugar. Opt for dried beans that you have to prepare yourself so you know there are no added ingredients.

Bottled Smoothies

Many brands of bottled smoothies have more sugar than soda and the misleading factor is their labels are allowed to say "no added sugars." This is because the sugar technically comes from fruit; however, when several pieces of fruit are processed, stripping nutrients, and condensed into a bottle, your body cannot decipher this type of sugar from the type found in a candy bar. Smoothies are a part of the keto nutrition plan, but opt for ingredients such as coconut milk, kefir, avocado, hemp seeds, kale, and berries.

"Fiber-Filled" Whole Wheat Bread and Pasta

The daily recommended fiber requirement is 25 grams for women and 38 grams for men. Excellent marketing by the food industry has made people believe that whole wheat bread, whole wheat pasta, and whole grain cereal are good sources of fiber. The truth of the matter is that you can get much more fiber per calorie in other sources of non-processed, natural foods. Below we compare different food sources of fiber, and illustrate how much one must eat of a particular food to obtain 30 grams of fiber.

Food	Calories Consumed to Reach 30 Grams of Fiber	Carbohydrates Consumed to Reach 30 Grams of Fiber	Sodium Consumed to Reach 30 Grams of Fiber
Whole Wheat Bread	1,350	270g	2025mg
Multi-Grain Cereal	1,275	275g	2300mg
Whole Wheat Pasta	1,260	246g	20mg
Avocado	702	36g	30mg
Flax Seed	550	30g	30mg
Strawberries	486	117g	6mg
Broccoli	465	90g	450mg
Kale	396	72g	300mg
Chia Seeds	385	33g	13mg
Raspberries	240	56g	4mg
Artichoke Hearts	195	45g	200mg

In addition to having more fiber per calorie, natural foods such as avocado, flax seeds, strawberries, broccoli, kale, chia seeds, raspberries, and artichokes are non-processed and contain no artificial additives but most commercially-made breads, pastas, and cereals do. Whole foods are superior when it comes to vitamins and minerals, too. Breads and cereals are fortified with vitamins, which means they do not occur naturally and are therefore harder to absorb. The next time you are in a grocery store, look at the ingredient labels of breads, pastas, and cereals—you'll find a plethora of ingredients (such as sugar, high fructose corn syrup, and preservatives) that are not ideal for weight loss, blood sugar, and overall wellness.

Cow's Milk

Once again, the marketing for milk has been genius—it does a body good, right? Well, not so much. First of all, cow's milk has hormones in it which help to grow very large cows! Even if you choose the organic brands, the hormones (intended for cows) still remain. Milk is touted for its calcium content and is known for building strong bones, but some studies suggest that calcium found in cow's milk has no correlation with strong bones and prevention of fractures.[5] Not to mention, at 12 grams of sugar per cup, it's not the ideal beverage for weight loss and blood sugar levels. For more beneficial sources of calcium, please refer to the table below.

Food	Serving	Calories	Calcium (Mg)	Sugar (G)
Sardines	3.5 ounces	210	351	0
Sesame seeds	¼ cup	206	351	0
Collard greens (cooked)	1 cup	49	300	1
Spinach (cooked)	1 cup	41	245	1
Canned salmon	4 ounces	155	232	0
Fresh wild salmon	6 ounces	300	120	0
Kale (raw)	1 cup	33	101	0
Almonds	23 almonds	162	75	1
Broccoli	1 cup	31	74	1.5
Butternut squash	1 cup	63	67	3

You will receive a lot of advice (good and bad) when it comes to nutrition—hopefully, we have cleared up some confusion for you by dispelling some of these popular "health food" myths. Nutrition can be complicated due to the never-ending and conflicting resources that are available in books and on the internet today. Many aspects of nutrition science have come from funded studies by special interest groups, so it is always best to scratch beneath the surface of popular recommendations and do your own research.

---

5   D. Feskanich et al., "Milk, dietary calcium, and bone fractures in women: a 12-year prospective study," NCBI, June 1997, accessed September 11, 2017, https://www.ncbi.nlm.nih.gov/pmc/articles/PMC1380936/.

Chapter 21

Super Simple Breakfast Recipes

Your *Super Simple Keto* recipes have six ingredients or less. If you happen to see a recipe with an extra ingredient or two, it may contain one of these kitchen essentials. These are important to have on hand and will not be counted toward the maximum of six total ingredients.

Salt

Pepper

Oil

Butter

Garlic (granulated or cloves)

Water

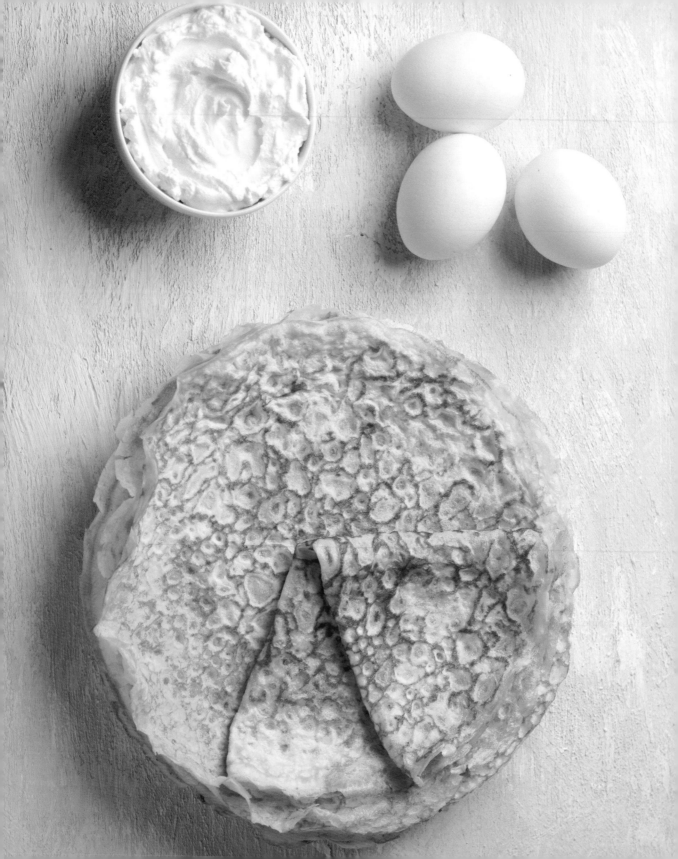

Keto Pancakes

These crepe-like pancakes are a favorite in the keto community and they are very low in carbohydrates and sugar. You can top them with berries, nut butters, bacon crumbles and butter, or salmon and crème fraîche.

Serves 2

½ cup cream cheese,
   softened
3 large eggs
3 tablespoons almond flour
Pinch of salt (optional)
Pinch of cinnamon
   (optional)
Butter for cooking

1. Place all ingredients except the butter in a blender and blend for 1 minute.

2. Using butter, cook in a hot pan for 1 minute on each side.

Prosciutto Egg Cups

These egg cups can be made ahead of time and taken on the go for a delicious and keto-friendly breakfast. For an impressive breakfast or brunch, multiply these ingredients by six to fill a 12-muffin tin, and pair with mixed greens and sparkling mineral water. If prosciutto is not readily available to you, you can replace it with deli ham.

Serves 1 (2 egg cups)

2 eggs

1 scallion, thinly sliced

1 tablespoon unsweetened full-fat coconut milk

Pepper, to taste

1 teaspoon oil

2 large prosciutto slices, folded in half

1. Preheat oven to 350°F.

2. In a small bowl, beat the eggs and combine with scallions.

3. Mix in the coconut milk and add freshly ground pepper, to taste.

4. Using the oil, grease two muffin tin spaces, and line each cup with one folded prosciutto slice.

5. Using the egg mixture, fill each cup until ⅔ full.

6. Bake for 30 minutes, until eggs are cooked through.

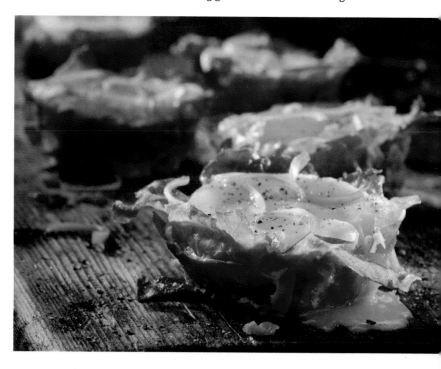

Eggs in a Hole

A low-carbohydrate take on the old classic, these eggs are encased in bell-pepper instead of high-glycemic bread. The bell peppers give a wonderful contrasting taste and texture to the eggs, and this dish pairs nicely with either tomatoes or fresh berries.

Serves 1

1 teaspoon extra-virgin olive oil

2½-inch sliced bell pepper rings

2 eggs

Salt and pepper, to taste

1. In a medium skillet, heat extra-virgin olive oil over medium heat.

2. Add bell pepper rings and sauté on one side for 2 minutes and then flip over.

3. Crack one egg into each of the bell pepper rings and reduce heat to low.

4. Cook the eggs through, about 10 minutes.

5. Add salt and pepper to taste, and serve warm, paired with tomatoes or berries.

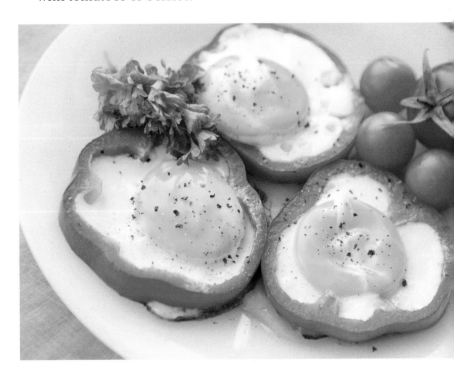

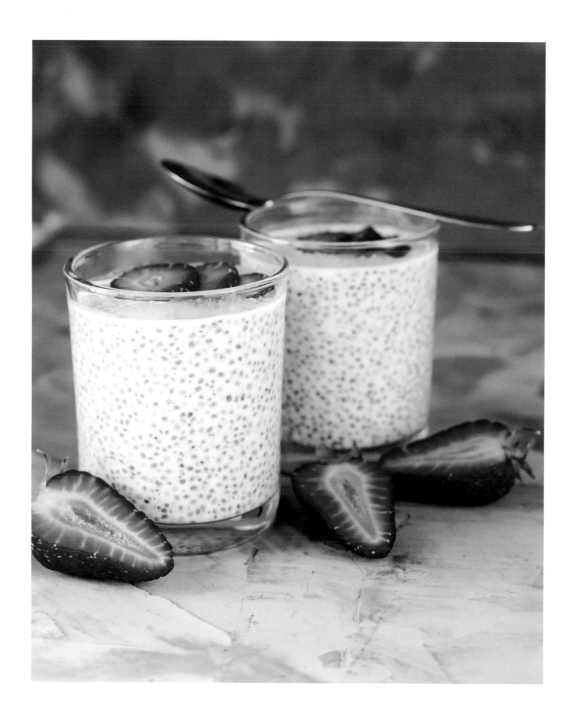

Easy Chia Seed Breakfast Pudding

This breakfast pudding only takes minutes to prepare and can be refrigerated overnight if you're looking for a quick and unique breakfast idea. If you need some added protein and fat, and like the combination of sweet and savory, simply pair with a slice or two of bacon.

Serves 1

½ cup unsweetened
  coconut milk
1½ tablespoons chia seeds
½ teaspoon vanilla extract
Fresh berries (optional)

1. Combine coconut milk, chia seeds, and vanilla extract in small bowl.

2. Cover and refrigerate for at least 2 hours, or overnight.

3. Top with your favorite berries (optional).

Pizza Eggs

Although this is a low-carbohydrate egg dish, each egg is dressed as its own mini pizza, and it's perfectly circular thanks to a mason jar lid. For added pizza topping flavor, use bell pepper rings (see page 173) instead of mason jar lids to encapsulate the eggs for a perfect mini pizza shape.

Serves 1

1 tablespoon oil, plus a
  little extra for greasing
2 large eggs
¼ cup Low-Sugar Pizza
  Sauce (page 246),
  divided
¼ cup shredded
  mozzarella, divided
10 mini pepperoni slices,
  divided
Freshly grated Parmesan,
  for garnish
Dried oregano, for garnish
Salt and pepper, to taste

1. Heat oil in medium skillet over medium heat, and grease the inner ring of two mason jar lids (to help the eggs keep a round shape). Place the rings from the jar lids in the center of the skillet and crack an egg inside each lid.

2. Top each egg with half of the pizza sauce, half of the cheese, and half the pepperoni slices.

3. Cover with a skillet lid and cook until egg whites have set and cheese has melted, 4 to 5 minutes.

4. Top with Parmesan and oregano, season with salt and pepper, and serve.

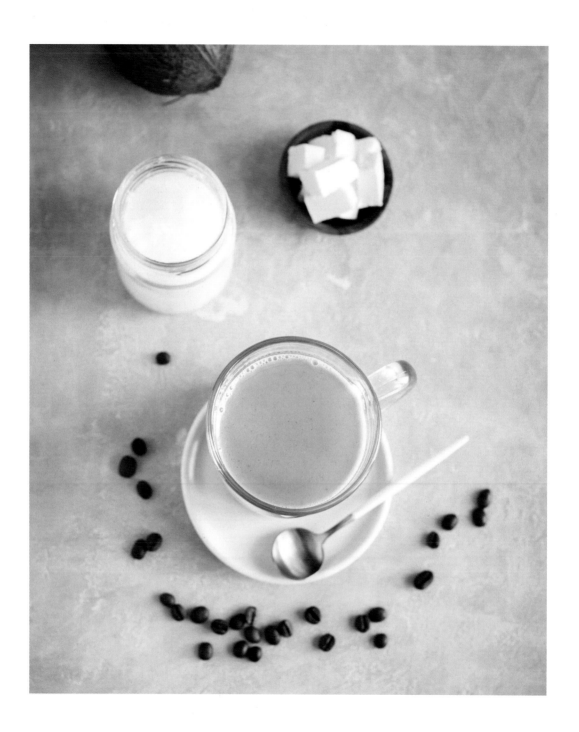

Keto Coffee

Keto coffee is calorie dense and will give you what you need for energy in the morning, even if you don't have time to prepare a traditional breakfast. If you're feeling like something more, pair with two eggs and sliced tomatoes, but this filling coffee can stand on its own!

Serves 1

8 ounces brewed, hot coffee
½ cup unsweetened almond milk or unsweetened coconut milk, heated
1 tablespoon butter or ghee
1 tablespoon MCT oil

1. Add all ingredients in blender, and blend for 15 seconds until frothy.

Turnip and Bacon Breakfast Hash

Breakfast hash is typically made with potatoes but you can use turnips to get the same potato texture and taste without all of the carbohydrates. This dish is filling enough on its own or you can choose to add two poached eggs on top for added protein and healthy fat.

Serves 2

1 tablespoon oil
1 large turnip, peeled and diced
Any seasoning of choice, to taste
¼ onion, diced
1 cup Brussels sprouts, halved
3 slices bacon
¼ cup red bell pepper, diced
Salt and pepper, to taste
1 tablespoon parsley for garnish

1. Add the oil to a large skillet over medium-high heat.

2. Add in the turnips and spices; cook 5 to 7 minutes, stirring occasionally.

3. Add in the onion and Brussels sprouts and cook 3 minutes, until they start to soften.

4. Chop the bacon into small pieces and add to the skillet, along with red bell pepper. Salt and pepper to taste.

5. Continue to cook another 5 to 7 minutes until the bacon is cooked. Garnish with parsley before serving.

No-Egg Breakfast Bake

Finding egg alternatives for your keto breakfast can changes things up and add variety to your nutrition plan. You may not commonly find breakfast casserole dishes that are egg-free, but they work well for a hearty breakfast. This breakfast bake pairs nicely with sliced tomatoes drizzled in olive oil and your favorite seasonings.

Serves 4

2 tablespoons oil, divided

2 large bell peppers of any colors, chopped

Any seasonings of choice, to taste

Salt and pepper, to taste

10 ounces pre-cooked turkey or pork breakfast sausage links of your choice

¾ cup grated mozzarella cheese

1. Preheat oven to 450°F.

2. Use ½ tablespoon oil to grease a medium-sized baking dish.

3. Place peppers into the baking dish, toss with 1 tablespoon oil and sprinkle with seasoning, salt, and pepper, and put the dish in the oven and bake 20 minutes.

4. While the peppers cook, heat the rest of the olive oil in a nonstick pan, add the sausages, and cook over medium-high heat until browned on all sides, about 10 to 12 minutes.

5. Remove the sausages and cut into thirds. Once the peppers have cooked for 20 minutes, add the sausages to the dish and bake for an additional 5 minutes.

6. Remove from oven and turn the oven to broil. Sprinkle the grated cheese over the sausage-pepper combination and put back in oven and broil 1 to 2 minutes, or until the cheese is nicely melted and starting to brown. Serve hot.

Five-Minute Coffee Cup Biscuits

These fluffy biscuits are made from keto-approved ingredients and only take a few minutes to make. Our favorite way to enjoy these is topped with butter or ghee, paired with fresh strawberries, or topped with cream cheese and lox.

Serves 2 (4 biscuits)

1 large egg
3 tablespoons almond flour
1 tablespoon coconut flour
1 tablespoon soft butter
1 tablespoon avocado oil
¼ teaspoon baking powder
Pinch of salt

1. Using a fork, thoroughly combine all ingredients in a microwave-safe mug until the mixture is smooth. Using the back of a spoon, smooth out the top into an even surface.

2. Microwave for 1 minute (based on your microwave, you may have to slightly alter the time and experiment with high versus medium-high temperatures).

3. Using a potholder or thick cloth, remove the hot mug from the microwave. Cover with a plate and turn upside down, allowing the biscuit to slide out of the coffee cup. Slice into 4 even pieces.

4. Serve with butter or ghee, and sliced strawberries.

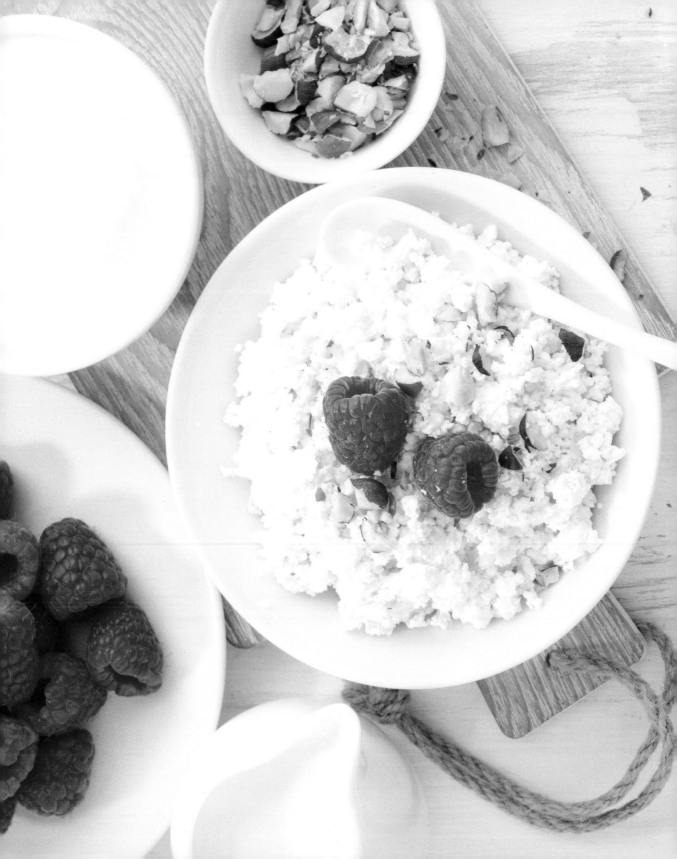

Cottage Cheese Breakfast Bowl

This recipe is super simple, but it's also super delicious and very filling. You only need five minutes to throw these ingredients together so it makes the perfect pre-work meal. Not to mention, it holds up well in the refrigerator so it can be packed the night before and taken on-the-go.

Serves 1

¾ cup cottage cheese

1 tablespoon hemp seeds

¼ cup fresh or frozen berries

2 tablespoons crushed almonds

1. Scoop the cottage cheese into a bowl, and top with hemp seeds, berries, and almonds.

Grain-Free Breakfast Granola

If you're looking for a cereal replacement that is devoid of grains and filled with protein and healthy fat, grain-free breakfast granola can be topped with your choice of nondairy milk or cream and berries. You'll have enough left over from this recipe to use the granola as a yogurt topping for another breakfast.

Serves 3 (½ cup per serving)

½ cup raw macadamia nuts, chopped

½ cup raw walnuts, chopped

¼ cup cacao nibs

2 tablespoons unsweetened coconut flakes

1 teaspoon vanilla extract

1 teaspoon ground cinnamon

¼ teaspoon salt

2 tablespoons coconut oil, melted

1. Preheat the oven to 325°F and line a baking sheet with parchment paper.

2. Combine the chopped macadamia nuts, walnuts, cacao nibs, coconut, vanilla, cinnamon, and salt in a medium bowl.

3. Add the coconut oil and mix well.

4. Spread the granola onto your prepared baking sheet and spread evenly into one layer.

5. Bake for 15 minutes or until the granola is toasted at the bottom and fragrant. Keep a close watch and stir frequently to prevent burning.

6. Let the granola cool and serve with your favorite nondairy milk.

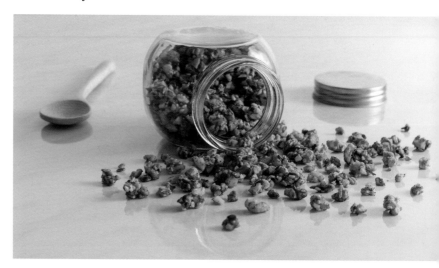

Breakfast Snack Pack

Sometimes you just don't have time to sit down to a hot breakfast so why not pack it to go? This easy-to-make egg and salmon breakfast box can be put together the night before a busy morning, and will ensure that you hit your keto macronutrients even on-the-go.

Serves 1

2 whole eggs
1 tablespoon oil
3–4 asparagus spears
2–3 ounces smoked salmon
1 slice cheese (optional)
Handful raw nuts
    (optional)

1. Bring 3 cups of water to a boil in a small pot. Once boiling, place the eggs in the pot; boil for 9 minutes for soft- to medium-boiled, or for 12 minutes for hard-boiled. Remove and run under cold water to stop the cooking process.

2. Meanwhile, sauté the asparagus in oil for 6 to 7 minutes or until tender and place in breakfast box.

3. Place the eggs, asparagus, and salmon in the meal containers. Add cheese and nuts (optional).

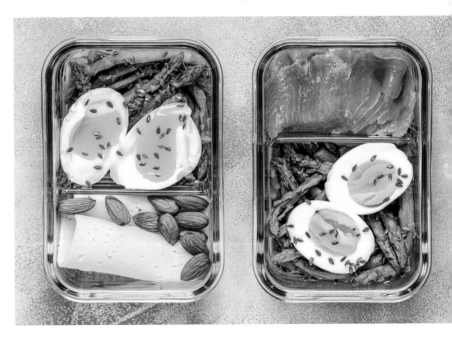

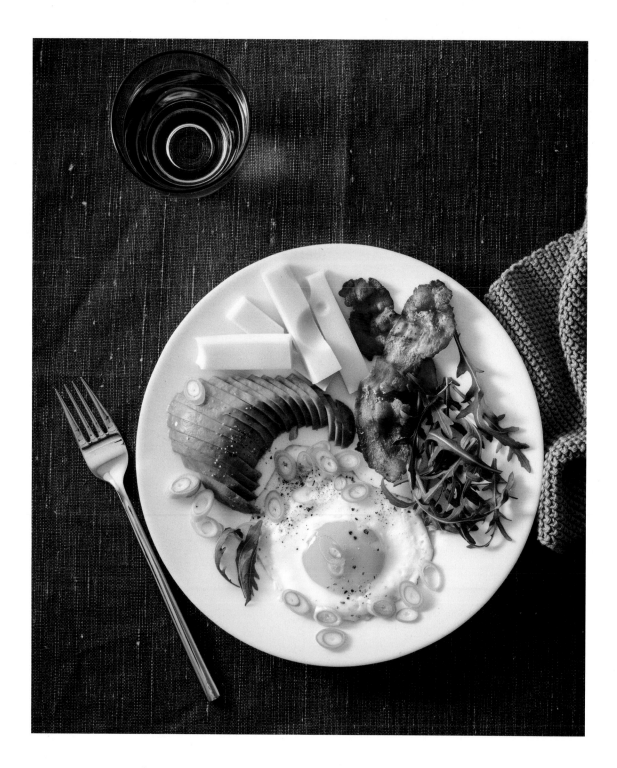

Bacon and Egg Platter

This dish is a bit more delectable and varied compared to the regular bacon and eggs breakfast. If you're cooking for a group, simply multiply the recipe and be sure to impress your friends if you're hosting a keto-friendly Sunday brunch. Garnishing with fresh arugula adds more vitamins and minerals, and complements the avocado.

Serves 1

2 pieces bacon
1 ounce cheese, sliced
½ avocado, sliced
Handful arugula
1 egg

1. Pan-cook bacon over medium-low heat, turning over every 2 minutes, until cooked through, about 10 minutes.

2. While the bacon is cooking, plate the cheese, avocado, and arugula.

3. Plate the bacon and add the egg to the hot bacon grease and cook through, about 5 minutes.

Cream Cheese and Lox Sliders

Your cream cheese and lox sliders can be made with just a few ingredients and in two completely different ways. If you're craving more of the traditional bagel with lox you would find in a deli, you can use the biscuits found on page 179. For a light and refreshing twist, opt for sliced cucumber in place of the biscuits.

Serves 2 (4 sliders)

4 Five-Minute Coffee Cup
   Biscuits (page 179)
3 ounces whipped cream
   cheese
3 ounces wild lox, chopped
Fresh dill, for garnish
Capers, for garnish
Freshly squeezed lemon, to
   taste

1. Spread equal amounts of cream cheese on each of the four biscuits.

2. Top each cream cheese biscuit with equal amounts of chopped lox.

3. Garnish each biscuit with fresh dill and capers, and top with a sprinkle of lemon juice.

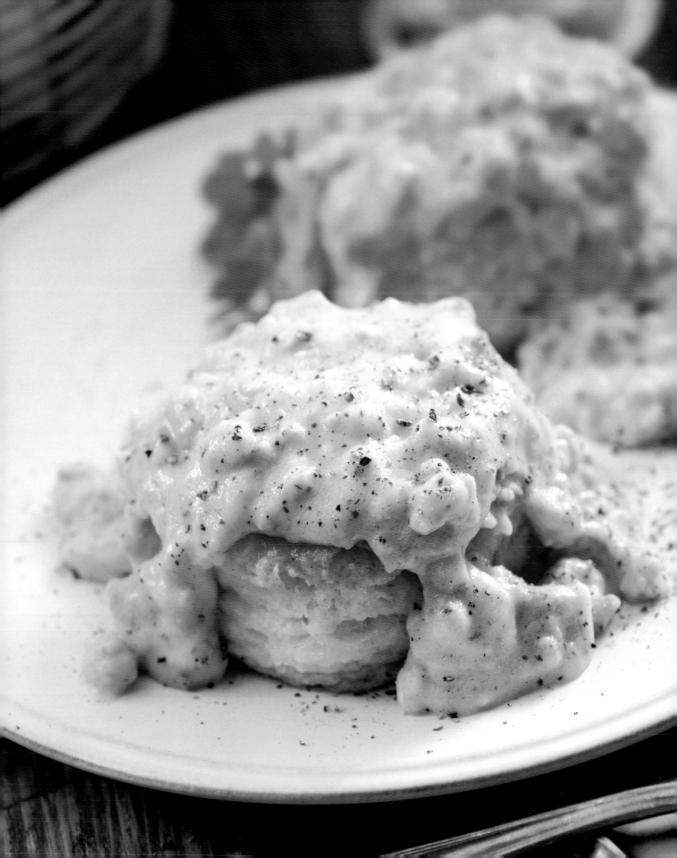

Biscuits and Gravy

Biscuits and gravy isn't a meal that is typically found on a keto breakfast menu, but with the Five-Minute Coffee Cup biscuits found in this chapter, you can still enjoy this country favorite. Feel free to pair your biscuits and gravy with eggs or fresh berries.

Serves 2

4 ounces breakfast sausage

3 ounces cream cheese, softened

⅓ cup half-and-half

Salt and pepper

4 Five-Minute Coffee Cup Biscuits (page 179)

Chopped fresh parsley for garnish (optional)

1. In a small saucepan over medium heat, brown the sausage while breaking into smaller chunks with a spatula.

2. Add the cream cheese and combine until blended.

3. Add the half-and-half and stir until thoroughly incorporated.

4. Let the gravy reduce over medium heat until you have reached a desired consistency, around 3 to 5 minutes. Remove from the heat and season with salt and pepper, to taste.

5. Pour the gravy over the biscuits and serve warm. Garnish with parsley, if desired.

Chapter 22

Super Simple Lunch Recipes

Your *Super Simple Keto* recipes have six ingredients or less. If you happen to see a recipe with an extra ingredient or two, it may contain one of these kitchen essentials. These are important to have on hand and will not be counted toward the maximum of six total ingredients.

Salt

Pepper

Oil

Butter

Garlic (granulated or cloves)

Water

Bell Pepper Nachos

Triangular bell pepper slices can be used as low-carbohydrate tortilla chips and with all of the nacho toppings, this dish tastes just like the classic. This base recipe can be modified to add any of your favorite nacho toppings and the flavors will be sure to quench any Mexican food cravings, and with zero guilt!

Serves 2–3

Oil for greasing
4 large bell peppers
   (assorted colors)
1 pound ground beef
3 tablespoons low-sugar
   taco seasoning
⅔ cup beef broth
1½ cups shredded cheese

Optional Toppings
½ cup diced tomatoes
⅓ cup diced green onions
½ cup mashed avocado
⅓ cup sour cream
Cilantro, to taste

1. Preheat oven to 375°F and grease a large baking sheet. Remove the membranes from the bell peppers and cut into triangle slices. Place on the sheet and bake for 10 minutes until tender.

2. While the peppers are roasting, brown the ground beef in a skillet over medium heat and drain the excess liquid.

3. Add the taco seasoning and beef broth and bring to a boil. Simmer over medium heat for about 5 minutes, or until it has reduced, leaving little to no liquid.

4. Spoon the ground beef on the bell pepper slices and top with shredded cheese. Return the baking sheet to the oven for 5 to 6 minutes, until the cheese has melted.

5. Remove from the oven and add the optional toppings of choice.

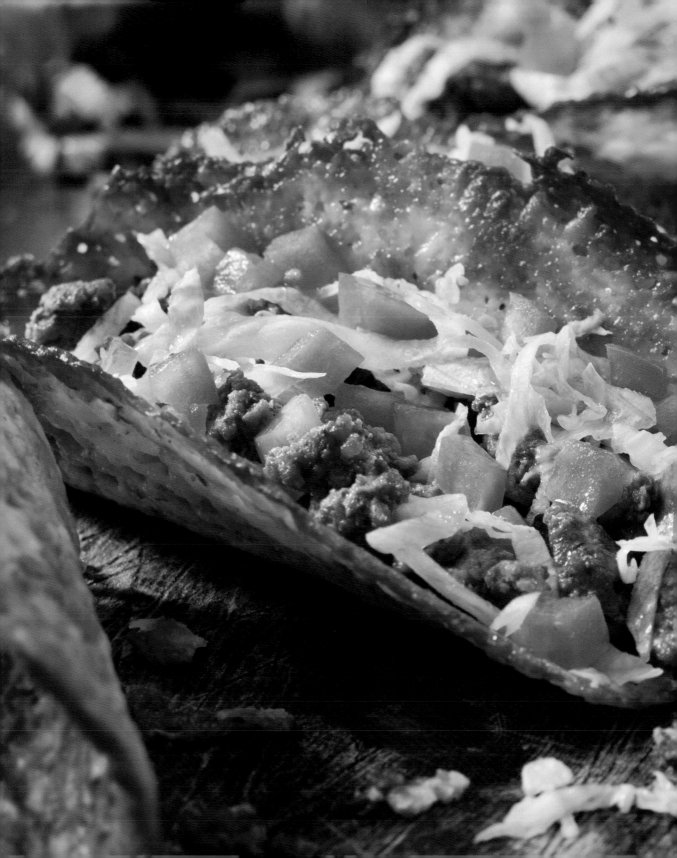

Cheese Shell Tacos

If you like your tacos with that crunchy chip-like shell, this dish is definitely for you. Just using one keto-approved ingredient (cheese) and a simple baking technique will give you crunchy taco shells with even more cheesy flavor. This base recipe is just the foundation for an array of possibilities for different proteins, sauces, seasonings, and toppings.

Makes 6 Tacos

2 cups shredded cheddar
    cheese
½ pound ground beef
1 tablespoon sugar-free
    taco seasoning
¼ cup water

Topping Suggestions
2 cups shredded lettuce
1 medium tomato, diced
⅓ cup diced yellow onions
1 avocado, sliced or mashed
½ cup sour cream
Fresh cilantro, to taste

1. Preheat the oven to 375°F and line two baking sheets with parchment paper.

2. Arrange the shredded cheese into 6 piles on the parchment-lined baking sheet, with plenty of space in between so the shells do not run together.

3. Bake or 7 to 10 minutes, until the edges start to brown and the cheese is no longer runny.

4. Meanwhile, prop up one wooden spoon or two kabob skewers (spaced 1 inch apart) with two cups or cans.

5. Remove the melted cheese rounds from the oven and while the cheese is still flexible, drape the cheese over the wooden spoon handle or skewers, letting it harden until cool. Repeat the process with all cheese rounds.

6. In a medium skillet, brown the ground beef, and drain the fat. Add the taco seasoning and water, stirring well. Bring to a simmer, and reduce for 3 to 5 minutes.

7. Remove ground beef from the heat and fill each cheese shell. Garnish with toppings of choice.

Spicy Mayo Ahi Poke Bowl

Preparing a sashimi-inspired dish at home can seem intimidating, but it's actually super simple. The key is to find high-quality and fresh sushi-grade fish, so check your local health food grocery that has a reputable seafood counter. After that, it's just a matter of chopping and mixing a few ingredients.

Serves 2

½ pound sushi-grade ahi tuna or salmon, cubed

¼ cup mayonnaise

1 tablespoon Sriracha sauce

1 avocado, cubed

¼ cup green onions, sliced

1 tablespoon black and/or white sesame seeds

1. Place the tuna in a medium-sized mixing bowl.

2. Combine the mayonnaise and Sriracha sauce to make the spicy mayo. Pour over the tuna and gently toss to coat.

3. Add the rest of the ingredients and gently toss to combine. Serve cold.

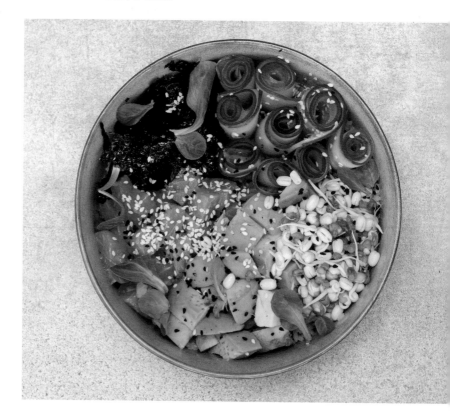

Pistachio Avocado Salad

This salad does well on its own, but if you're looking for more protein, chicken is a great addition. The fats from nuts, seeds, avocado, and oil will help you hit your keto macros in the healthiest way possible. If you prefer to batch prepare this so you have several servings for the week, simply sub kale in for the romaine as it stands up better after a few days in the fridge.

Serves 2

For the Salad

1 head romaine lettuce, chopped

3 green onions, chopped, or ¼ cup sliced red onions

½ cup shelled pistachio halves

¼ cup shelled hemp seeds

1 avocado, diced

For the Dressing

2 tablespoons extra-virgin olive oil

1 tablespoon apple cider vinegar

1 tablespoon coconut aminos

Freshly squeezed lemon, to taste

1. Place the chopped lettuce in a large bowl.

2. Add the green onions, pistachios, hemp seeds, and avocado.

3. Whisk all dressing ingredients and thoroughly toss in the salad.

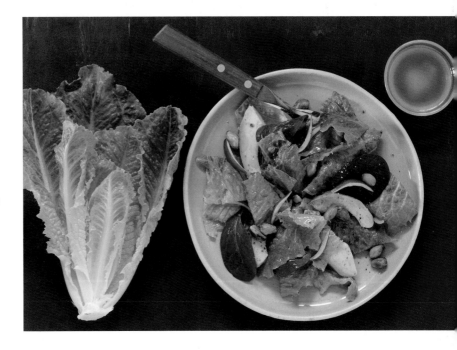

Easy Lunchtime Roasted Cheesy Chicken

Sometimes we just don't have time to prepare a nice roasted chicken dish for lunch but this recipe is so easy, you can whip it up in only five minutes. Not to mention, the flavors are unique to most poultry dishes so it's not only simple, but also different. Pair this decadent fare with a simple side salad or your favorite roasted veggies for a complete meal.

Serves 4

½ cup grated or shredded Parmesan cheese
1 cup mayonnaise
1 teaspoon garlic powder
1½ teaspoons salt
½ teaspoon pepper
4 chicken breasts

1. Preheat oven to 375°F. Line a baking sheet with aluminum foil or parchment paper.

2. Excluding the chicken breasts, combine all other ingredients in a medium bowl.

3. Using a spoon, spread the mixture over the chicken breasts.

4. Bake for 45 minutes, and serve warm.

Lunch Snack Pack

Sometimes you don't feel like an actual meal for lunch and a variety of delicious snacks will do the trick—not to mention, it can be easier and faster to pack and take on-the-go. For a full week of lunches, simply multiply this recipe by five, package, and refrigerate as it will all hold up for the week.

Serves 1

1 small container Greek yogurt
4 strawberries
¼ cup raw walnuts
Handful of raw broccoli florets and celery sticks
½ cup mashed avocado for dipping
2 tablespoons peanut butter for dipping
1 hard-boiled egg

1. Package all ingredients in a portable container and refrigerate.

British Bangers and Mash

Although we do advise limiting processed meats, if you're in a pickle for a quick lunch, this is a great option. Not to mention, I thought I would pay homage to my British roots with this one! A tip is to quadruple the mashed cauliflower recipe so you have the tasty low-carb side dish on-hand in your refrigerator.

Serves 1

1 cup cauliflower florets
2 hot dogs or sausages
¼ cup grated Parmesan
   cheese
Salt and pepper, to taste
Mustard, to garnish
   (optional)
Sauerkraut, to garnish
   (optional)

1. Steam the cauliflower over medium-high heat until extremely tender, about 20 minutes.

2. Meanwhile, prepare the hot dogs or sausages according to package directions.

3. Once the cauliflower is steamed, mash it in a medium bowl with the grated Parmesan, salt, and pepper until thoroughly combined.

4. Plate the hot dogs or sausages with the mashed cauliflower and garnish (optional).

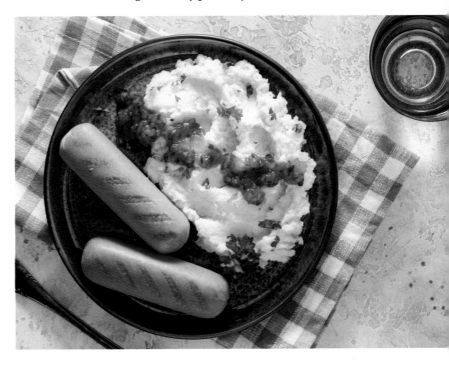

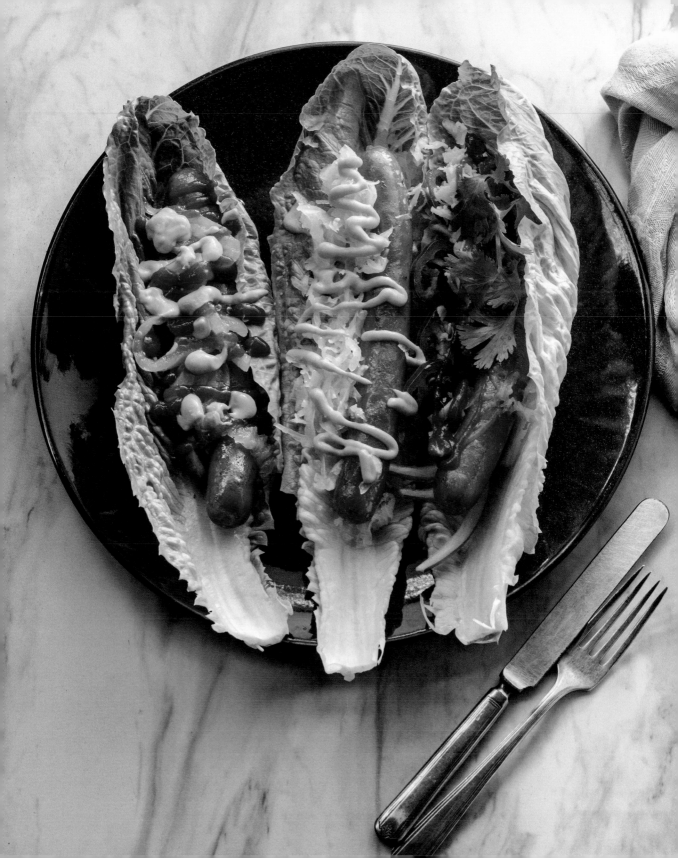

Keto Hot Dogs Your Way

We don't recommend too many meals of hot dogs (or deli meats) but once in a while it is *Super Simple Keto*-approved. This hot dog dish has a delicious combination of flavors, making your standard non-keto hot dog seem a bit boring. You won't even miss the bun!

Serves 1

2 nitrate-free hot dogs

2 large romaine lettuce leaves

2 tablespoons sauerkraut

1 tablespoon sliced red onion

2 tablespoons grated cheddar cheese

Ketchup and mustard, to taste

1. Grill or boil the hot dogs until warmed through.

2. Place each hot dog on a lettuce leaf.

3. Top one hot dog with sauerkraut and mustard.

4. Top the other hot dog with onion, cheese, ketchup, and mustard.

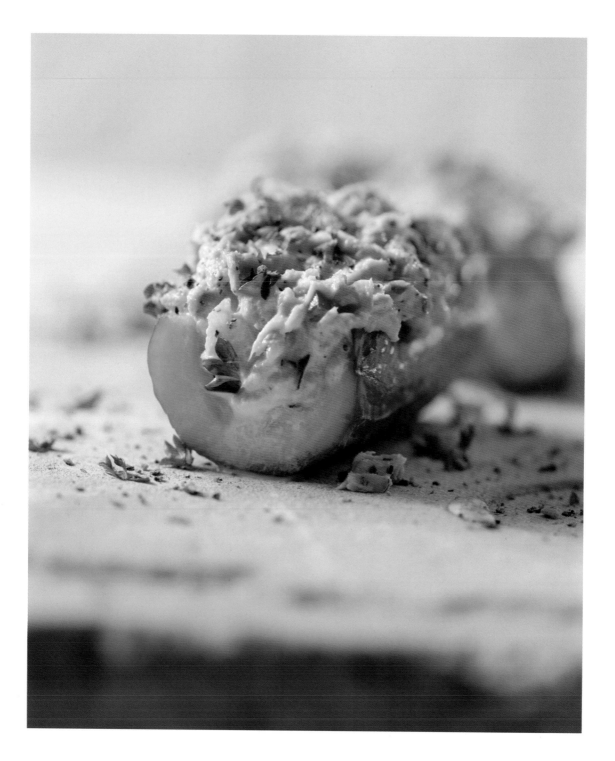

Zucchini Boat Tuna Salad

This is a healthier version of traditional mayo-filled tuna salad and the hand-held zucchini boats make them convenient for a picnic or work lunch. This simple recipe is high protein, high healthy fat, and low-carbohydrate, and only takes minutes to prepare.

Serves 1

1 large zucchini
1 can tuna packed in water (strain as much water out of can as possible)
1 tablespoon avocado oil mayo
Juice from ½ lemon
¼ bell pepper, diced
Handful of parsley, chopped
Black pepper, to taste

1. Halve the zucchini lengthwise, and hollow out by scraping out the inner soft layer and set aside.

2. Mix tuna with avocado oil mayo, lemon juice, and bell pepper.

3. Fill zucchini boat with tuna mixture and top with parsley and ground pepper.

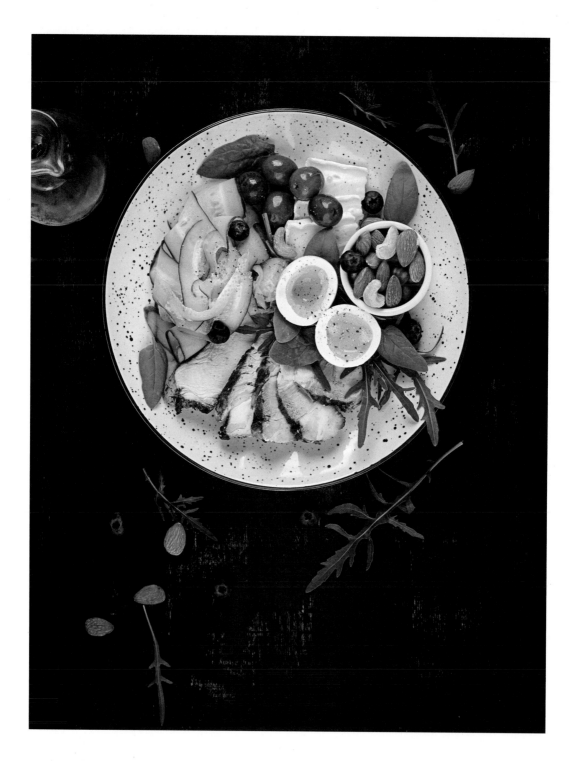

Wine Country Lunch Platter

Sometimes it's nice to change it up and have a smorgasbord platter as opposed to a standard hot meal. This is the perfect lunch to introduce your new keto lifestyle to your friends—and you can even enjoy a glass of red wine or two with it!

Serves 1

4 ounces cooked pork chop, sliced

½ cup chopped or sliced cucumber

1 egg, soft-boiled, halved

1 ounce cheese, sliced

5 olives

1 ounce nuts

¼ cup berries (optional)

1. Arrange all ingredients on a platter.

2. Serve with a glass of Pinot Noir or Sauvignon Blanc (optional).

Egg Roll in a Bowl

This dish gives you all of the delicious fillings found in a Chinese egg roll, in one big bowl. Since these bowls keep really well in the refrigerator, this is a great recipe to batch cook ahead of time so you have tasty Chinese-inspired food for the week.

Serves 2–3

1 pound ground chicken or pork sausage

1 teaspoon minced ginger

3 tablespoons soy sauce

1½ teaspoons sesame oil

4½ cups packaged coleslaw mix (shredded cabbage and carrots)

3 green onions, chopped

1. Brown the meat in a medium nonstick skillet until cooked all the way through and then add the ginger, soy sauce, and sesame oil.

2. Add the coleslaw and stir until coated with sauce.

3. Add chopped green onions, mix thoroughly.

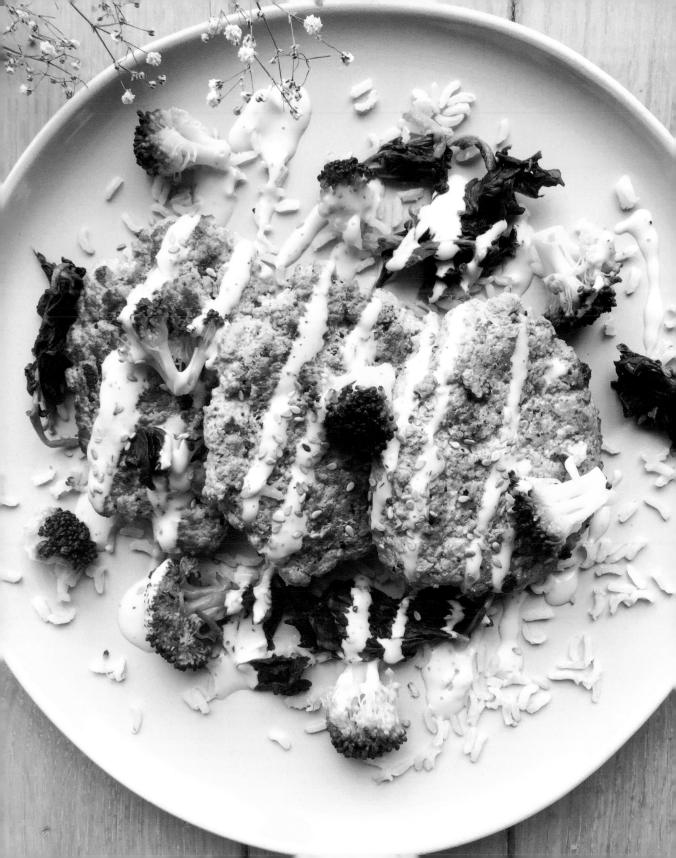

Tuna Burgers

Crab cakes are delicious, but let's face it—they can be expensive and difficult to make. These easy (and inexpensive!) tuna burgers are reminiscent of your favorite seafood restaurant's crab cakes but can be made in a snap and with ingredients found in the kitchen cupboard. Avocado oil mayonnaise and whole grain mustard make great keto-friendly dips for your tuna burgers.

Serves 4

2 (5-ounce) cans solid white albacore in oil

2½ tablespoons almond flour

2 tablespoons mayonnaise

1 large egg, beaten

Salt and pepper, to taste

½ tablespoon olive oil or avocado oil

Optional:

Chopped scallions, to taste

Capers, to taste

1. In a medium bowl, combine all ingredients (including optional ingredients, if using), except the oil. Mix until thoroughly combined.

2. Form the mixture into 4 patties, around ¾-inch thick.

3. In a large pan, heat the oil over medium-high heat. Place the patties in the pan.

4. Cook the patties on one side for 4 to 5 minutes, or until they have set and the undersides are golden.

5. Flip the patties over and cook for 4 to 5 minutes.

6. Serve warm, or store in the refrigerator in an airtight container with parchment paper to separate the patties.

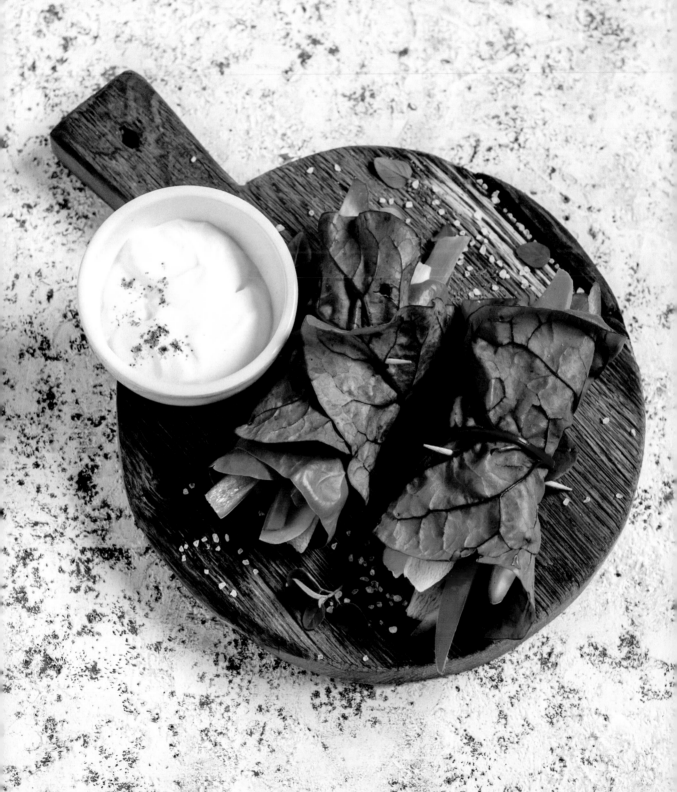

Mediterranean Swiss Chard Wrap

This low-carb wrap is a refreshing change of pace! This base recipe can be added to with lots of colorful produce and dipping sauces. Or if you are looking for more protein, diced chicken or steak makes a tasty addition.

Serves 1

2 tablespoons full-fat plain yogurt

2 tablespoons crumbled feta cheese

2 tablespoons pitted, chopped olives

¼ ripe avocado, diced

Salt and pepper, to taste

2 large Swiss chard leaves

4 thin slices bell pepper (any colors)

1. In a large bowl, mash the yogurt, feta, olives, and avocado into a chunky paste. Season with salt and pepper and set aside.

2. Place the Swiss chard leaves on a cutting board and using a knife, remove the stems and around 2 inches of the spine from each leaf.

3. Divide the yogurt mixture in half and spoon into each leaf. Place the sliced bell pepper on the mixture and roll into a wrap. Secure with a toothpick.

4. To form a burrito-style wrap, place a horizontal mound of mixture on the lower third of each leaf, just above the area where the spine was removed, and add the bell pepper slices. Fold in the two vertical ends of one leaf and roll from the bottom. Secure with a toothpick.

5. Repeat with the second wrap and enjoy cold.

Parmesan Kale Salad

This universal salad base will accommodate your favorite toppings of choice as it pairs nicely with most foods and flavors. The avocado dressing is simple and healthy, and provides a creamy texture that is reminiscent of more decadent salad dressings that sometimes don't have the most ideal ingredients. Diced hard-boiled eggs or chopped steak are complimentary additions.

Serves 1

2 cups curly kale or chopped romaine
½ avocado
2 tablespoons oil
1 teaspoon apple cider vinegar
1–2 tablespoons grated Parmesan cheese
Freshly squeezed lemon, to taste

1. Place the curly kale or romaine in a medium bowl.

2. In a small bowl, mash the avocado with a fork until you have a paste-type of texture.

3. Drizzle in the oil gradually and thoroughly combine with the avocado.

4. Drizzle in the apple cider vinegar and thoroughly combine with the avocado mixture.

5. Using your hands, massage the avocado dressing into the kale or lettuce until all leaves are coated.

6. Top with Parmesan cheese, and freshly squeezed lemon, to taste.

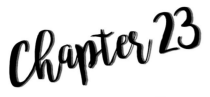

Super Simple
Dinner Recipes

Your *Super Simple Keto* recipes have six ingredients or less. If you happen to see a recipe with an extra ingredient or two, it may contain one of these kitchen essentials. These are important to have on hand and will not be counted toward the maximum of six total ingredients.

Salt

Pepper

Oil

Butter

Garlic (granulated or cloves)

Water

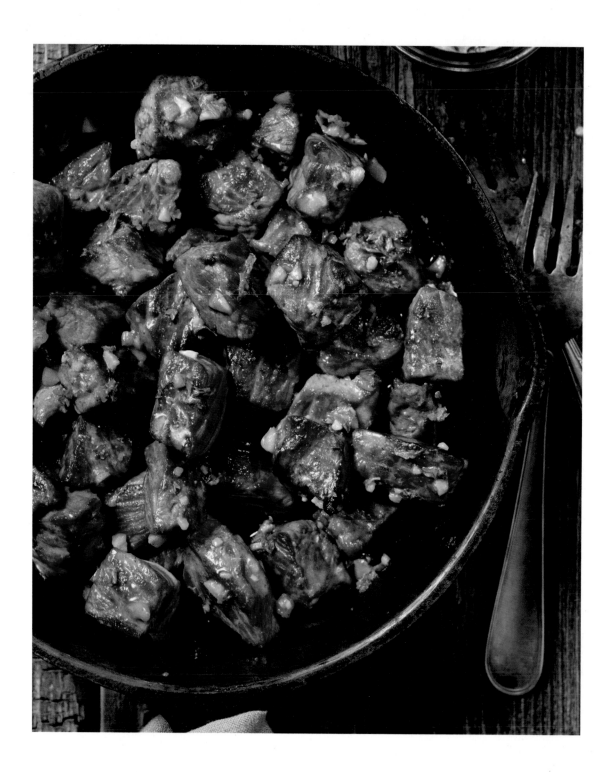

Garlic Butter Steak Bites

This is a unique and simple way to prepare your steak, and so many variations can be created from this easy base recipe by adding your own seasonings and flavors. Steak bites are delicious with a trio of dips—mashed avocado, Avocado Oil Mayo (page 250), and Tzatziki (page 249) are our favorites, or you can pair with a side salad with ranch dressing.

Serves 3-4

2 pounds ribeye steak
Salt and pepper, to taste
4 tablespoons oil, divided
4 tablespoons butter, divided
2 large cloves garlic, minced and divided
1 teaspoon fresh parsley leaves, minced

1. Cut steak into ¾-inch cubes and season with salt and pepper.

2. Heat half of the oil in a large skillet over medium-high heat. Add half the steak in a single layer and cook, turning a few times until golden and medium rare, about 5 minutes.

3. Add half of the butter and half of the garlic and toss to coat.

4. Remove steak to a serving bowl. Repeat with remaining steak.

5. Garnish with parsley.

Rosemary Goat Cheese and Mushroom Stuffed Pork Chops

If you're looking for a pork chop dish that is a bit more fancy and flavorful, but doesn't require lots of ingredients, this meal can be used for an easy dinner at home or even to host a gathering. For a pop of flavor, pair the stuffed chops with some crisp sauerkraut.

Serves 2

½ cup chopped white mushrooms

2 ounces goat cheese, crumbled

1 teaspoon rosemary, freshly chopped or dried

1 large clove garlic, pressed

2 (12-ounce) bone-in pork chops (1-inch thick)

Salt and pepper, to taste

1 tablespoon oil

1. Preheat oven to 350°F.

2. In a small bowl, gently mix the mushrooms, goat cheese, rosemary, and garlic.

3. Cut a large slit in the side of each pork chop to make a pocket for the filling. Do not pierce the back or sides of the chops so the filling doesn't spill out.

4. Stuff the pork chops with the goat cheese filling, and press closed. Season the pork chops with salt and pepper, to taste.

5. Heat the oil in a large oven-safe skillet over medium-high heat. Add the stuffed chops and sear until golden brown, 2 to 3 minutes per side.

6. Transfer the skillet to the oven and cook for 25 to 30 minutes, until the internal temperature of the chops reaches 145°F. Allow them to rest for 3 minutes before serving.

Au Gratin Radishes

Your favorite potatoes au gratin can be recreated in the keto way by substituting potatoes with radishes. Radishes are extremely low in carbohydrates but can mimic the potato texture, especially when prepared in a creamy cheese sauce. This recipe serves as an excellent base but you can use any additions you like such as cooked chicken, ground beef, or bacon.

Serves 4-6

3 tablespoons butter

½ large yellow onion, finely chopped

1 cup heavy whipping cream

⅓ cup Parmesan cheese, shredded

1 cup cheddar cheese, shredded

Salt and pepper, to taste

5 cups sliced radishes

Chopped scallions, for garnish

1. Preheat oven to 350°F.

2. In a medium pot, melt the butter over low heat.

3. Add the onions and let cook until slightly tender, around 3 minutes.

4. Add the heavy whipping cream and let simmer for 4 to 5 more minutes, stirring occasionally.

5. Slowly add all of the cheese, stirring continuously, to melt into a smooth, creamy mixture.

6. Salt and pepper to taste and stir.

7. Remove from heat, and grease an 8- or 9-inch square baking pan.

8. Layer with radishes to cover the bottom. If you are using additional ingredients like bacon or cooked chicken, add them on top of the radishes. Add some of the melted cheese mixture.

9. Repeat step 8 until you are out of radishes and melted cheese, and bake for 1 hour. Once cooked, garnish with scallions.

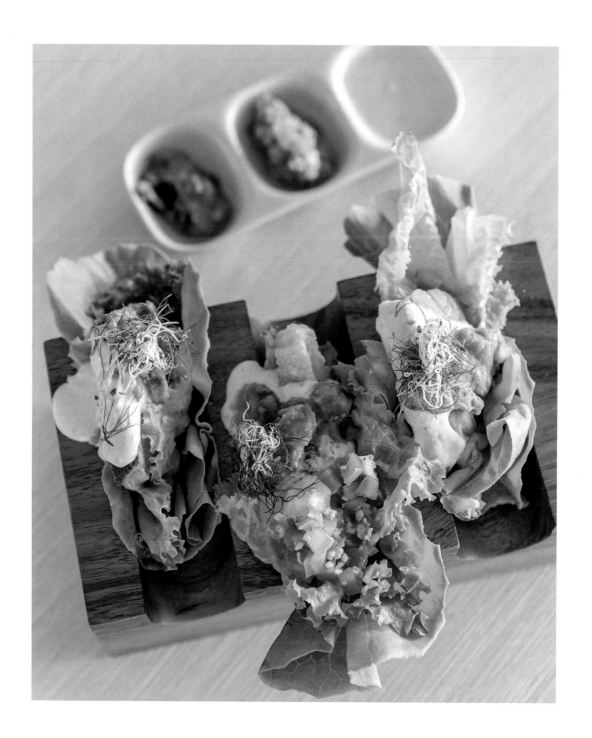

Simple Salmon Taco Lettuce Wraps

This simple recipe is light and refreshing but filled with flavor. Reminiscent of traditional seaside Mexican cuisine, the healthy fats will keep you satisfied while the low-glycemic carbohydrates will provide antioxidants and fiber. Brighten these wraps up by squeezing fresh lime on top.

Serves 2

1 tablespoon oil
1 pound salmon
Salt and pepper, to taste
1 head butter lettuce
1 avocado, mashed
2 tablespoons Greek yogurt
2 tablespoons pico de gallo
    or salsa
1 lemon, cut in half

1. Heat the oil in a medium pan and add the salmon.

2. Add salt and pepper to taste, and cook over medium heat until cooked through. Break the salmon apart while cooking—leaving the skin on or removing is optional.

3. Layer the lettuce, mashed avocado, Greek yogurt, salsa, and lemon.

4. Assemble the tacos by scooping the cooked salmon into individual lettuce cups and topping with taco add-ons, and freshly squeezed lemon.

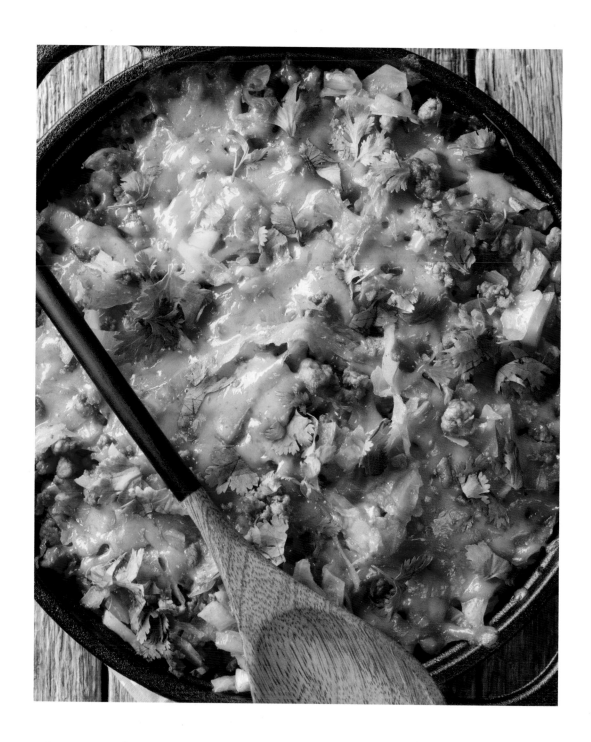

Cheesy Beef Cabbage Roll Casserole

This is a casserole take on the classic cabbage roll dish, but it has some added cheese for a rich and creamy texture. To batch cook, simply double, triple, or even quadruple this recipe as this casserole is freezer friendly. Serve warm with a small arugula salad.

Serves 4–5

2 pounds ground beef
4 cups cabbage, shredded
½ yellow onion, thinly sliced
¾ cup sour cream
2 teaspoons garlic powder
Salt and pepper, to taste
1 cup shredded cheddar cheese, divided
Cilantro for garnish (optional)

1. Preheat oven to 400°F.

2. In large pan over medium-high heat, brown the ground beef, while breaking into pieces with a spatula for 3 to 4 minutes.

3. Add the cabbage and onion and combine; continue to cook for 5 to 6 minutes while stirring and breaking up the beef.

4. Remove from heat and add in sour cream, stirring until combined. Add the garlic powder, salt, pepper, and half of the shredded cheddar cheese while mixing.

5. Pour into a baking dish and bake for 30 minutes. Top with the remainder of the shredded cheese and return to the oven until cheese is melted and browned, around 5 minutes. Garnish with cilantro (optional).

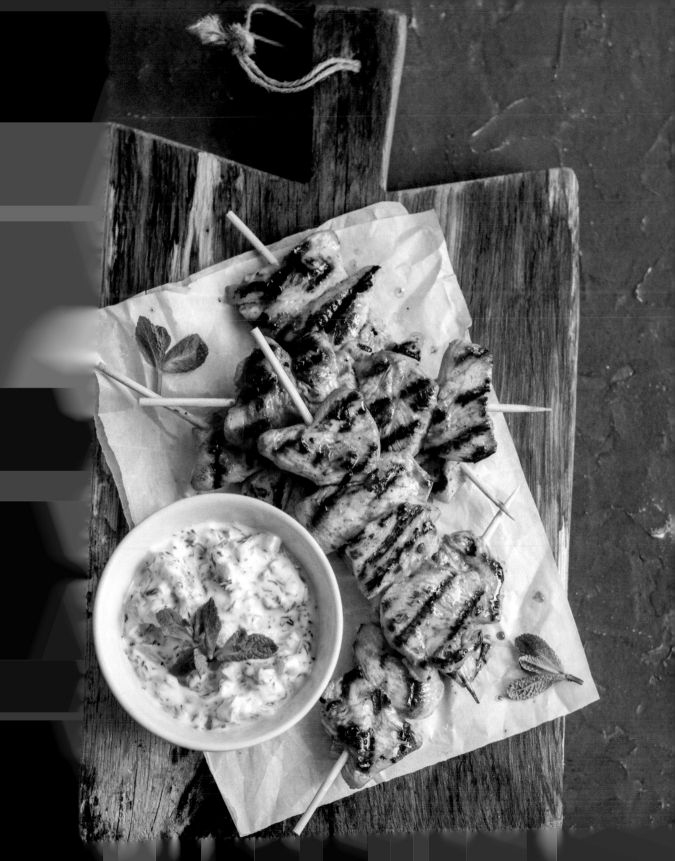

Spiced Chicken Skewers with Tahini-Yogurt Dip

This keto-approved dish will satisfy your Indian food cravings without the use of any rice or legumes. If you're unfamiliar with the spice, garam masala is used in a variety of curry and lentil dishes, and can be found in many mainstream grocery stores. If you're in a red meat mood, simply replace the chicken with steak.

Serves 3

1 cup plain Greek yogurt
¼ cup chopped fresh parsley
¼ cup tahini
2 tablespoons lemon juice
1 clove garlic
¾ teaspoon salt, divided
1 tablespoon oil
2 teaspoons garam masala
1 pound boneless/skinless chicken breasts, cut into 1-inch pieces

1. Prepare you grill with nonstick cooking spray for direct cooking or preheat your broiler.

2. For the tahini-yogurt dip, combine yogurt, parsley, tahini, lemon juice, garlic, and ¼ teaspoon salt in a food processor or blender; process until combined and set aside.

3. Combine oil, garam masala and remaining salt in a medium bowl. Add chicken and toss to evenly coat. Thread the chicken on 8 (6-inch) metal or wooden skewers.

4. Grill chicken skewers over medium-high heat or broil 5 minutes per side or until chicken is no longer pink. Serve with tahini-yogurt dip.

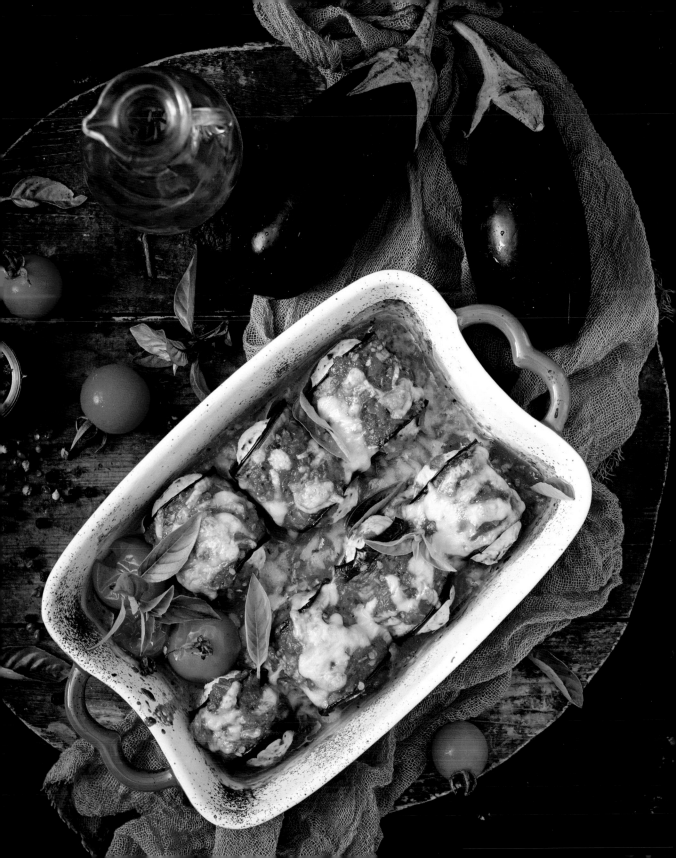

Italian Eggplant Roll-Ups

If you're craving a keto-friendly lasagna, this dish has all of the elements but is far less labor-intensive. These roll-ups are just the base of endless opportunities—other ingredients such as spicy sausage and bell peppers make wonderful additions. Pair with a crisp Caesar salad for an Italian keto experience without the carbohydrates.

Serves 6

1 large eggplant

Salt and pepper, to taste

1 cup cottage cheese or ricotta cheese

½ cup shredded mozzarella cheese

Garlic powder, to taste

1 teaspoon Italian seasoning mix

½ cup low-sugar marinara sauce, divided

1. With the stem side up, stand the eggplant and cut it lengthwise into ¼-inch slices, for a total of around six portions.

2. Rub both sides of each eggplant slice with salt and pepper, to taste.

3. Place the eggplant slices on a layer of paper towels and allow them to "sweat" for 15 minutes to remove excess moisture.

4. Preheat the oven to 350°F.

5. Pat the eggplant dry with fresh paper towels and transfer the slices to a rimmed baking sheet.

6. Bake the eggplant until it is barely tender, about 15 minutes. Be sure not to overcook it.

7. While the eggplant slices are in the oven, combine the cottage cheese, mozzarella, salt and pepper, garlic powder, and Italian seasoning in a medium bowl.

8. Remove the eggplant from the oven and allow them to cool for 5 minutes.

9. Raise the oven temperature to 400°F.

10. Spoon ¼ cup of the marinara sauce into the bottom of a 13x9-inch baking dish.

11. Spoon 2 tablespoons of the cottage cheese mixture onto an eggplant slice. Roll it up and place it seam-side down on the marinara sauce in the baking dish. Repeat until all slices have been filled, folded, and placed.

12. Top the roll-ups with the remaining marinara sauce and bake for 20 minutes.

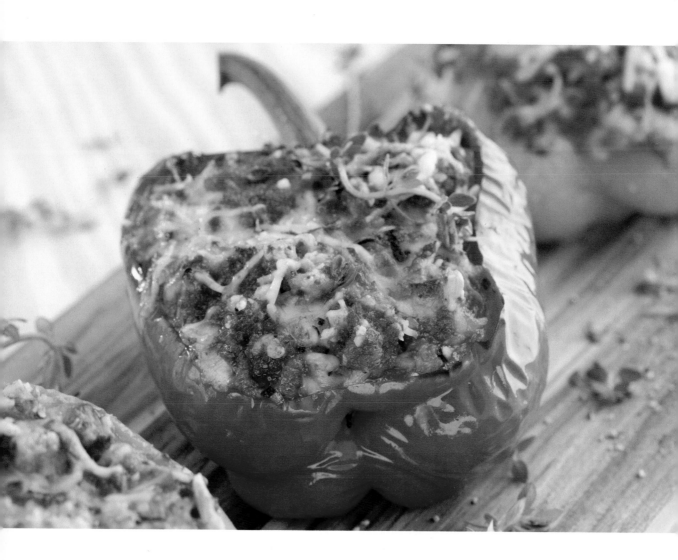

Keto Stuffed Peppers

Stuffed peppers are the quintessential comfort food and are still hearty without the rice. This dish can be made in larger batches ahead of time and reheated for a keto meal on-the-go. Stuffed peppers are a complete dish on their own or can be paired with an arugula salad.

Serves 2

1 cup riced cauliflower

1 tablespoon oil

1 teaspoon dried oregano, divided

Salt and pepper, to taste

6 ounces Italian sweet or hot sausage, casing removed

½ cup grated provolone cheese, divided

2 large red bell peppers

1. Preheat oven to 350°F.

2. Place the cauliflower rice, oil, half the oregano, salt, and pepper in a large sauté pan over medium heat. Cover the pan to steam until tender, about 6 minutes. Remove the pan from heat and set aside.

3. In another pan, cook the sausage (while breaking it apart), remaining oregano, salt and pepper, until the sausage is no longer pink, around 8 minutes. Set the pan aside.

4. Add the sausage, the fat from the pan, and the cauliflower rice to a large bowl with ¼ cup of the cheese. Stir to combine and adjust seasonings if necessary, and set the bowl aside.

5. Cut the bell peppers lengthwise and remove membranes. Place the peppers cut side up into a baking dish and spoon the sausage mixture into each pepper half. Top with a sprinkle of cheese.

6. Cover the dish with foil and bake for 25 minutes. Remove the foil and bake for 10 more minutes, or until the cheese is bubbly.

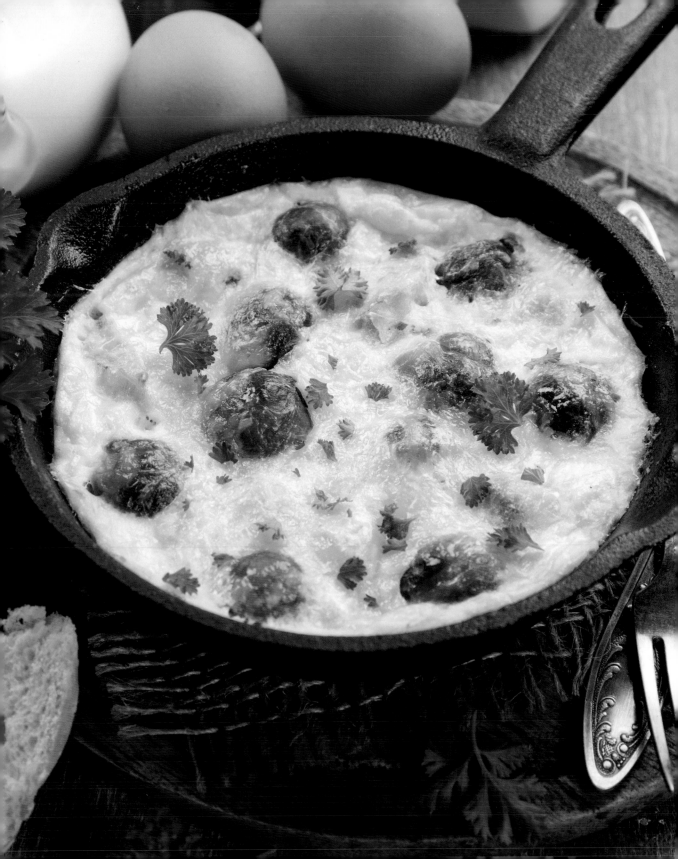

Creamy Brussels Skillet Casserole

Even if you don't like Brussels sprouts, you will love them this way. This creamy and cheesy dish stands up on its own or you can use this recipe as a base, adding chicken or salmon. This casserole can be prepared ahead of time as it keeps well in the refrigerator, and can be easily reheated.

Serves 4

6 ounces bacon, chopped

2 pounds Brussels sprouts, trimmed and halved

2 cloves garlic, minced

1½ cups heavy cream

1 tablespoon lemon juice

½ cup shredded Parmesan cheese

Salt and pepper, to taste

1. Place a large deep skillet over medium heat. Add the bacon and cook until browned. Remove the bacon to a plate, keeping the bacon fat in the pan.

2. Add the Brussels sprouts to the bacon fat and cover the pan. Cook until tender, stirring occasionally, around 8 to 9 minutes.

3. Add the garlic and stir for 1 minute until fragrant. Add the heavy cream and bring to a simmer.

4. Stir in the lemon juice and then sprinkle the top with the Parmesan cheese, and stir to combine.

5. Season with salt and pepper, bring to a simmer, and then remove from heat. Garnish with reserved bacon.

Spinach, Artichoke, Asparagus Stuffed Chicken

This is a favorite of many keto dieters, and it's a very family-friendly way to get some veggies in the meal. For an interesting seafood dish, just follow the same instructions but use two thick salmon fillets instead of chicken. This is a complete keto meal, or it can be served with a crisp side salad.

Serves 2

2 chicken breasts

4 tablespoons store-bought spinach artichoke dip, divided

6 asparagus spears

Salt and pepper, to taste

1. Preheat the oven to 350°F.

2. Butterfly the chicken breasts and spread 2 tablespoons of spinach artichoke dip on each butterflied breast.

3. Add 3 asparagus to each breast.

4. Fold the dip- and asparagus-filled chicken back into one whole breast and secure with cooking twine.

5. Season with salt and pepper and bake for 35 minutes.

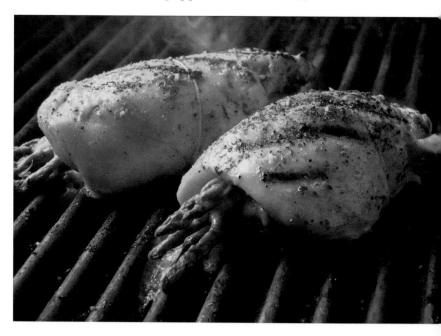

Bunless Philly Cheesesteaks

The flavor in a good Philly cheesesteak lies in the steak, onions, peppers, and melting provolone, so you won't miss the bun in this dish. If you're looking for some keto-friendly bread to stack this decadent mixture on, a sandwich chaffle found in chapter 13 will surely do.

Serves 2

1 tablespoon butter
1 cup white mushrooms
½ cup chopped onions
⅓ cup chopped green bell pepper
½ teaspoon garlic powder
8 ounces rare roast beef slices
2 slices provolone cheese
Salt and pepper, to taste

1. In a medium-sized pan over medium heat, melt the butter and then add the mushrooms, onions, bell peppers, and garlic powder. Cook until the vegetables are soft, about 4 to 5 minutes.

2. Slice the roast beef into strips or 1-inch squares.

3. Add the roast beef to the pan and toss with the produce mixture for 1 minute, until heated through.

4. Reduce the heat to low and top the roast beef mixture with the provolone cheese. Cover the pan with a lid and continue to heat for 2 to 3 minutes, until the cheese is melted. Season with salt and pepper, to taste.

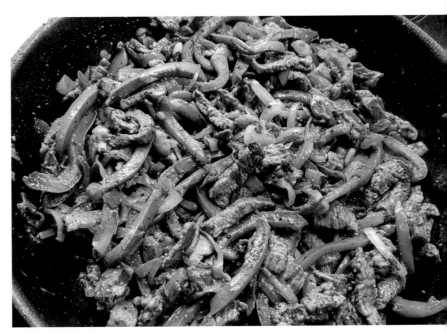

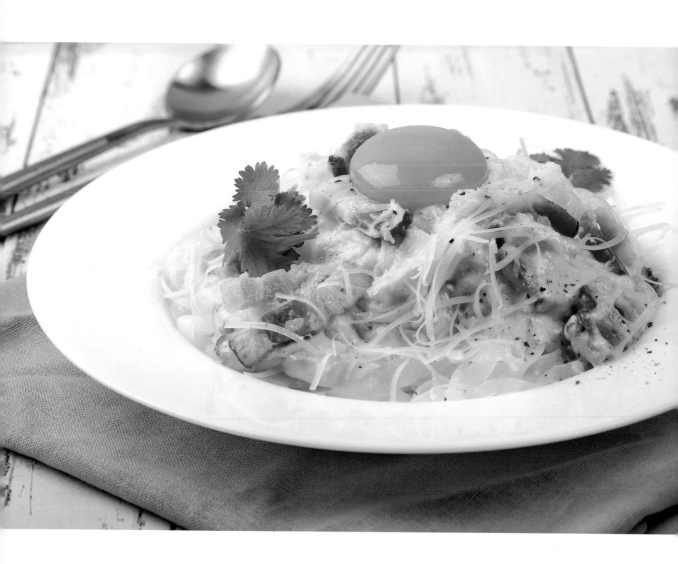

Shirataki Carbonara

This carbonara rendition is a keto-revised take on the old classic. Even if your family isn't following the same keto plan, they will be sure to love this rich and creamy pasta dish. If you can't find Shirataki noodles at your local grocery store, zoodles (zucchini noodles) work well as a substitution.

Serves 2

4 slices bacon

3 ounces chicken breast, chopped

1 (7-ounce) packet Shirataki noodles

1 large egg yolk

2–3 tablespoons Parmesan cheese

1 cup heavy whipping cream, divided

1. Dice the bacon and cook over medium heat until it changes color but does not get crispy. Remove from pan and set aside.

2. Cook the chopped chicken pieces over medium heat in the same pan as the bacon, until almost fully cooked, around 6 minutes. Remove the chicken and set aside.

3. Meanwhile, dry fry (using a dry frying pan with no oil or butter) the Shirataki noodles so that all excess water evaporates, around 7 minutes.

4. In a small bowl, thoroughly combine the egg yolk and Parmesan cheese until you have a smooth paste.

5. In the same pan used for the bacon and chicken, add half of the cream and the Parmesan egg mixture and combine over medium heat. This may take a few minutes until it is smooth.

6. Add the remaining cream, chicken, and bacon and incorporate.

7. Combine the chicken bacon sauce with the noodles and serve hot.

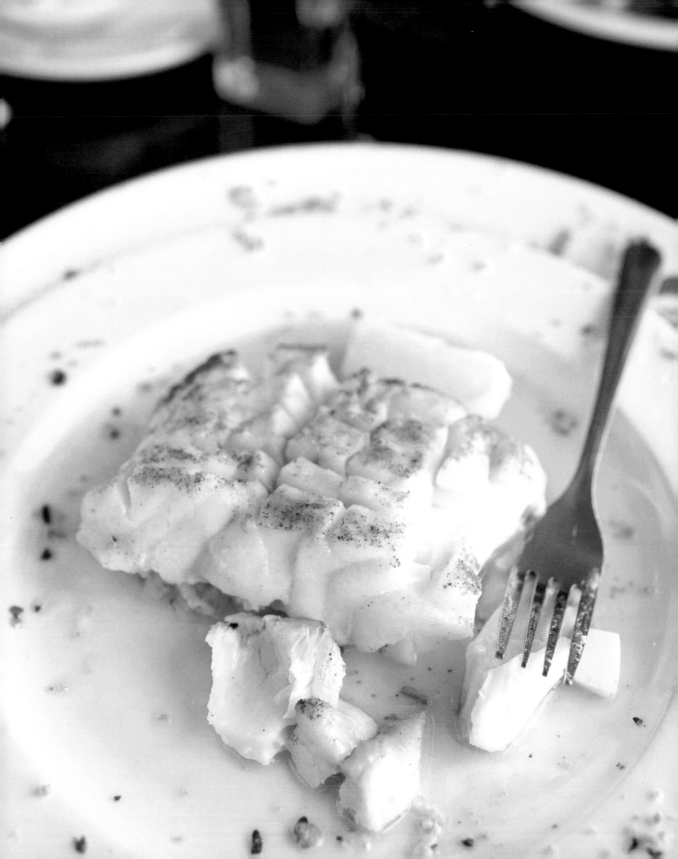

Easy Bake Lemon Butter Fish

If you are newer to seafood, this is a wonderful recipe to try as it has a very mild fish taste—if you like chicken, you will probably enjoy this dish! Mild white fish pairs well with steamed or sautéed green beans, with a generous amount of freshly squeezed lemon on top. To brighten it up even more, add some more fresh herbs in addition to the parsley.

Serves 4

¼ cup melted butter
4 cloves garlic, minced
Zest and juice of 1 lemon,
 plus 1 lemon sliced
2 tablespoons minced fresh
 parsley
Salt and pepper, to taste
4 filets of cod, halibut, or
 rockfish

1. Preheat oven to 425°F.

2. In a bowl, combine the butter, garlic, lemon zest and juice, and parsley; season with salt and pepper to taste.

3. Place the fish in a greased baking dish.

4. Pour the lemon butter mixture over the fish and top with fresh lemon slices.

5. Bake for 12 to 15 minutes, or until fish is flaky and cooked through.

6. Serve the fish topped with fresh parsley and freshly squeezed lemon juice.

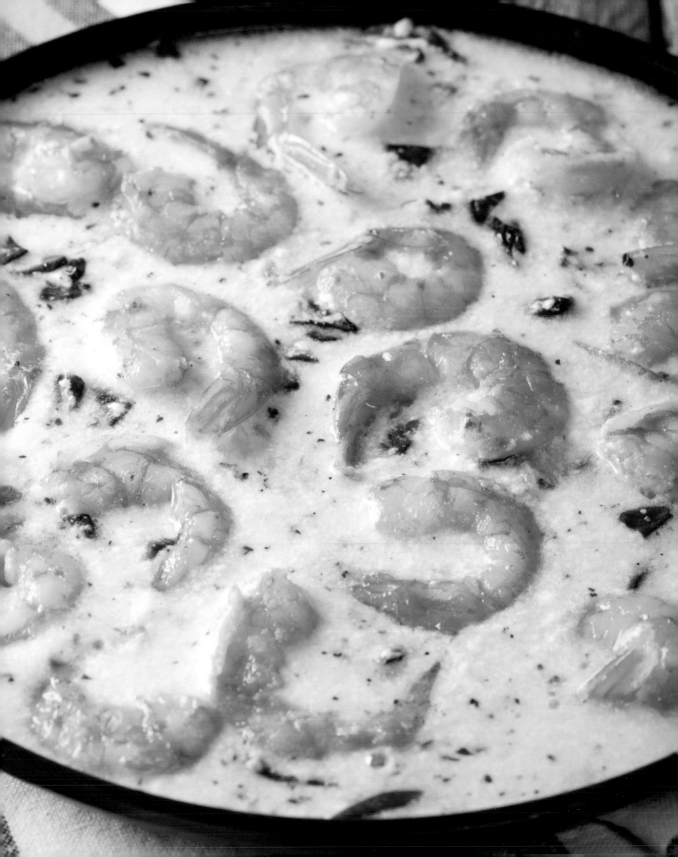

Creamy Tuscan Shrimp

If you're not a fan of shellfish, this recipe works just as well with chicken. This dish pairs well with a crisp salad or can be poured over riced cauliflower for an even heartier meal.

Serves 3–4

2 tablespoons olive oil

2 tablespoons butter

1 pound shrimp, deveined, and tails removed

Salt and pepper, to taste

3–4 cloves garlic, minced

1 cup halved cherry or grape tomatoes

3–4 cups baby spinach

¾ cup heavy cream

¼ cup freshly grated Parmesan

2 tablespoons basil, thinly sliced

1. Heat oil and butter in a large skillet over medium-high heat, until the oil is very hot and the butter has melted.

2. Carefully add the shrimp and sprinkle with salt and pepper; sauté for 1 minute on each side.

3. Remove the shrimp from pan and set aside. Add the garlic, tomatoes, and spinach to the same pan. Sauté until the garlic is fragrant, about 1 minute.

4. Stir in the heavy cream, Parmesan cheese, and basil and reduce heat to medium. Simmer until sauce is slightly reduced, about 2 to 3 minutes.

5. Return the shrimp to the pan and stir to combine. Serve warm.

Chapter 24

Super Simple Soups, Side Dishes, Snacks & Sauces

Your *Super Simple Keto* recipes have six ingredients or less. If you happen to see a recipe with an extra ingredient or two, it may contain one of these kitchen essentials. These are important to have on hand and will not be counted toward the maximum of six total ingredients.

Salt

Pepper

Oil

Butter

Garlic (granulated or cloves)

Water

Taco Soup

Serves 4–6

1 pound ground beef

3 tablespoons low-sugar taco seasoning, divided

4 cups beef bone broth (or any broth of choice), divided

2 (14.5-ounce) cans diced tomatoes (with liquid)

¾ cup ranch dressing

1. Brown the ground beef in a large pot over medium-high heat for 7 to 10 minutes, or until no longer pink. Drain if desired.

2. Add 2 tablespoons of the taco seasoning and ¾ cup of the broth. Simmer for 4 to 5 minutes, or until the liquid is mostly gone.

3. Add the remaining broth, diced tomatoes (with liquid), and the remaining tablespoon of taco seasoning, and combine.

4. Bring to a low boil and simmer for 8 to 10 minutes, and remove from heat.

5. Wait 2 minutes and then stir in the ranch dressing. Add any desired garnishes such as sour cream, green onions, cheddar cheese, cilantro, or avocado.

Creamy Spinach Soup

Serves 4-6

3 cups raw spinach

3 cloves garlic, minced

2 tablespoons butter or ghee

1½ cups bone broth or vegetable broth

1 cup heavy whipping cream

1 cup shredded mozzarella cheese (optional)

1. Over medium heat in a large pan, sauté the spinach and garlic in butter until the spinach is wilted, around 5 minutes.

2. Add the bone broth and whipping cream and combine.

3. Transfer to a blender and blend for 2 to 3 minutes.

4. Transfer back to the pan and heat until the soup boils.

5. Add the mozzarella cheese and stir until melted (optional).

Cream of Mushroom Soup

Serves 4

1 tablespoon oil

½ large onion, diced

2½ cups mushrooms, sliced

6 cloves garlic, minced

2 cups chicken or vegetable broth

1 cup heavy cream

1 cup unsweetened almond milk

Salt and pepper, to taste

1. In a large pot over medium heat, sauté the onions and mushrooms in oil for about 10 to 15 minutes, stirring occasionally, until lightly browned. Add the garlic and sauté for 2 more minutes.

2. Add the chicken broth, cream, almond milk, salt, and black pepper. Bring to a boil, then simmer for 15 minutes, stirring occasionally.

3. Use an immersion blender to puree until smooth, or puree in batches in a regular blender.

Broccoli and Cheese Soup

Serves 4-6

1 tablespoon oil

4 cloves garlic, minced

3½ cups chicken broth (or vegetable or bone broth)

1 cup heavy cream

4 cups broccoli, chopped into small florets

3 cups cheddar cheese, divided

1. In a large pot over medium heat, add the oil and sauté garlic until fragrant, about 1 minute.

2. Add the chicken broth, heavy cream, and chopped broccoli. Increase heat to bring to a boil.

3. Once it begins to boil, reduce heat and simmer for 15 to 20 minutes, until broccoli is tender.

4. Add ½ cup of the cheddar cheese, simmer, and stir until melted. Repeat this process ½ cup at a time until all the cheese is used. Be sure to keep the heat at a very low simmer and avoid high heat, to prevent seizing.

5. Remove from heat immediately once all the cheese melts, and serve.

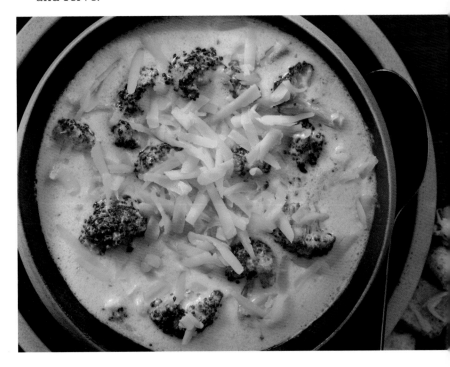

Chicken Vegetable Soup

Serves 4

2 tablespoons oil

1 medium onion, chopped

5 cloves garlic, smashed

3 cups riced cauliflower

¾ teaspoon crushed red
  pepper flakes

4 stalks celery, thinly sliced

6 cups low-sodium chicken
  broth or bone broth

2 boneless skinless chicken
  breasts

Salt and pepper, to taste

1. In a large pot over medium heat, heat the oil and add the onion and garlic. Cook until the onions and garlic begin to brown.

2. Add the riced cauliflower to the pot and cook over medium high heat until it begins to brown, about 8 minutes.

3. Add the red pepper flakes, celery, and chicken broth and bring to a simmer.

4. Add the chicken breasts and let cook slowly until they reach an internal temperature of 165°, about 15 minutes. Remove the chicken from the pot and shred once they are cool enough to handle. Meanwhile, continue simmering until vegetables are tender, 3 to 5 minutes more.

5. Add the shredded chicken back to soup, and season to taste with salt and pepper.

Bone Broth

Serves 4

1 gallon (4 liters) of water

2 tablespoons apple cider vinegar

2-4 pounds chicken or beef bones

Salt and pepper, to taste

1. Place all ingredients in a large pot or slow cooker.

2. Bring to a boil.

3. Reduce to a very low simmer and cook for 12 to 24 hours. The longer it cooks, the better it will taste and more nutritious it will be. If using a slow cooker, add all ingredients and cook on low for 12 to 24 hours.

4. Allow the broth to cool. Strain it into a large container and discard the solids.

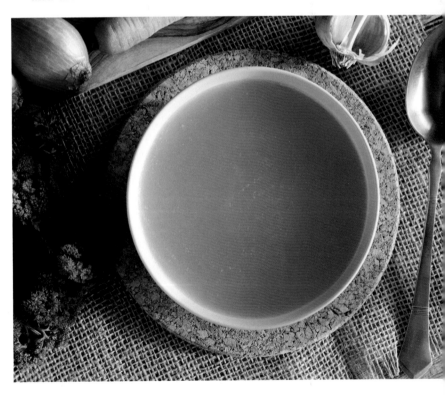

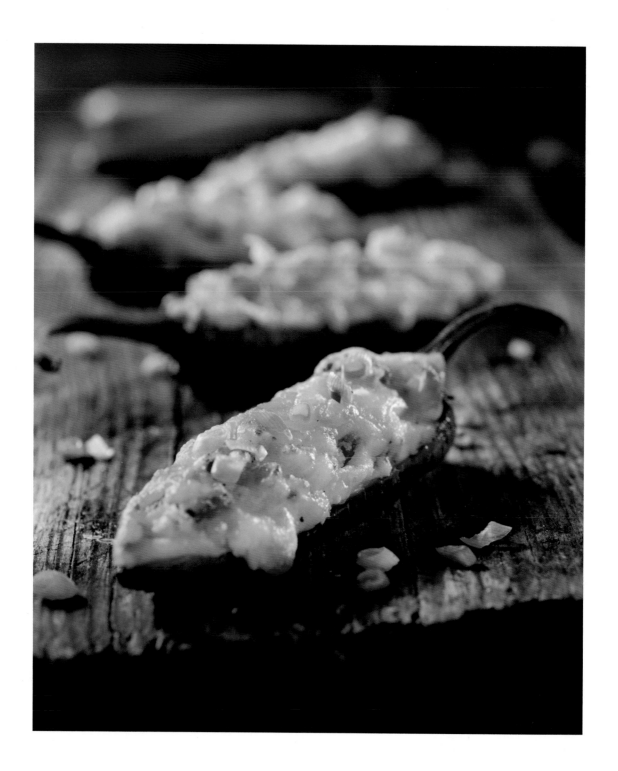

Jalapeño Poppers

Serves 3

5 slices bacon

6 jalapeño peppers

3 ounces cream cheese, softened

¼ cup shredded cheddar cheese

½ teaspoon garlic powder

1. Preheat oven to 400°F and line a baking sheet with parchment paper.

2. In pan over medium heat, cook the bacon until crispy, around 10 minutes, flipping over occasionally. Chop and set aside.

3. Slice the jalapeños in half lengthwise and remove inner seeds and membranes.

4. In a medium bowl combine the cream cheese, cheddar cheese, garlic powder, and cooked bacon.

5. Spoon the cheese mixture into each jalapeño half and set the filled peppers cheese side up on the lined baking sheet.

6. Bake for 18 to 20 minutes until the cheese is melted and slightly crisp on top.

Spinach Artichoke Dip

Makes 2 Cups

1 (9-ounce) box frozen spinach, defrosted

1 (14-ounce) can artichoke hearts

8 ounces cream cheese

¼ cup sour cream

1 teaspoon garlic powder

Salt and pepper, to taste

½ teaspoon red pepper flakes (optional)

1 cup mozzarella

1. Place defrosted spinach and artichokes in a colander and press firmly to extract as much liquid as possible, and set aside.

2. Add cream cheese to a medium microwave-safe bowl and soften in the microwave for 30 seconds or until the cream cheese is the same consistency as mayonnaise.

3. Add spinach, artichokes, sour cream, garlic powder, salt and pepper, and red pepper flakes (optional) and combine. Fold in the mozzarella cheese.

4. Refrigerate for at least one hour and serve with vegetables to dip or as a steak topper or baked salmon or chicken stuffer.

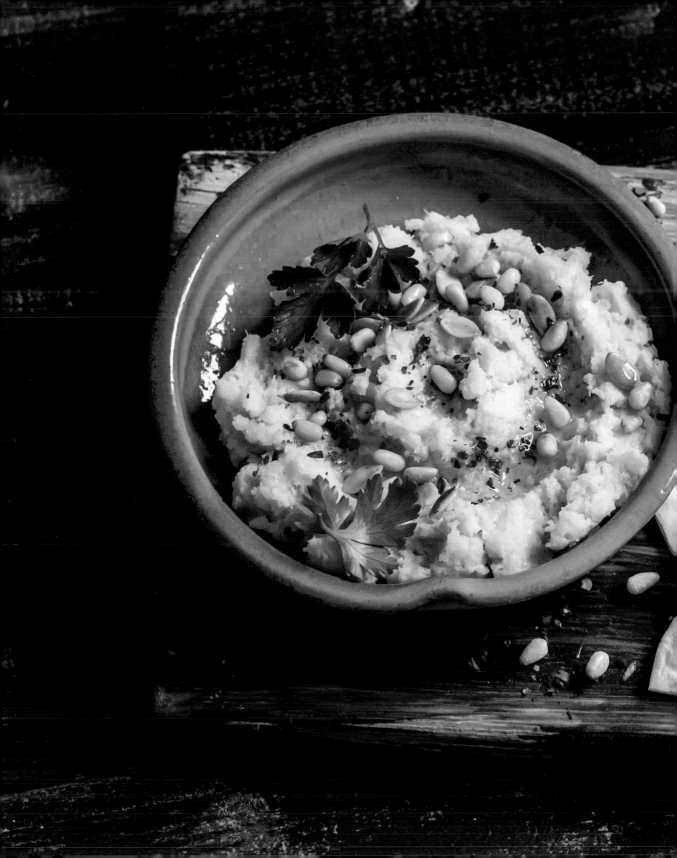

Cauliflower Hummus

Serves 4

1 medium head cauliflower
5 tablespoons extra-virgin
   olive oil, divided
½ cup tahini
2 cloves garlic
⅓ cup lemon juice
1 teaspoon salt
½ teaspoon ground black
   pepper
Chopped fresh parsley, to
   taste (optional)

1. Preheat oven to 375°F and chop cauliflower into small florets.

2. Toss cauliflower in 1 tablespoon of extra-virgin olive oil and place on a baking sheet; roast until tender, about 20 minutes.

3. Place the roasted cauliflower in a food processor or blender and combine with the other 4 tablespoons of oil, and the rest of the ingredients.

Four-Ingredient Salmon Dip

Makes 2 Cups

8 ounces smoked salmon,
   finely chopped
8 ounces crème fraîche
Juice from 2 lemons
1–2 tablespoons fresh dill,
   finely chopped

1. In a medium bowl, combine the salmon and crème fraîche until the crème fraîche turns pink.

2. Add the lemon juice and dill and mix until thoroughly incorporated.

3. Serve with endive leaves or radish slices to dip.

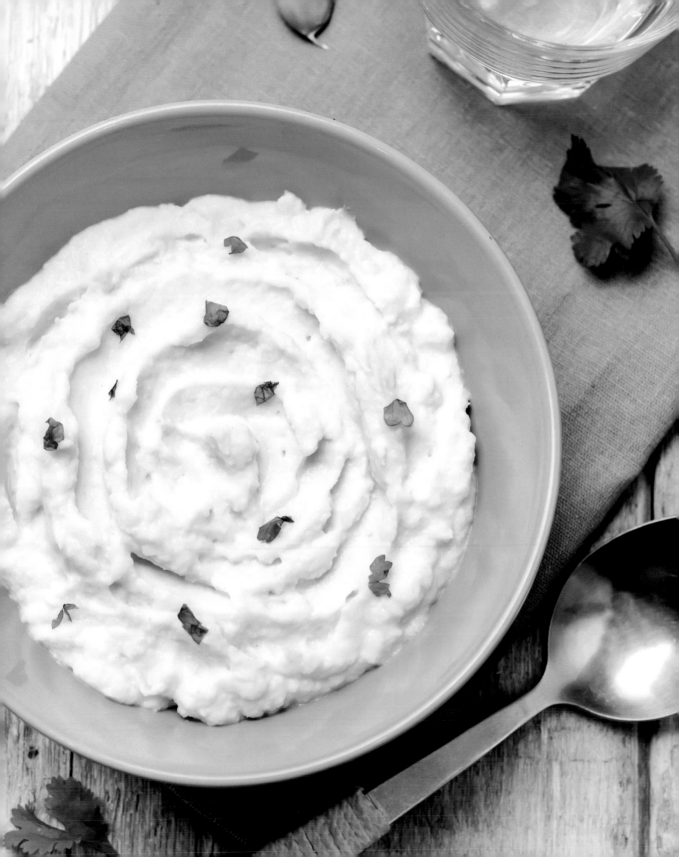

Mashed Cauliflower

Serves 4

1 head of cauliflower
½ cup grated Parmesan
  cheese

1. Chop cauliflower and steam until extremely tender.

2. Using a potato masher or fork, mash into a mashed potato-like texture.

3. Add grated Parmesan and thoroughly combine.

Parmesan Roasted Fennel

Serves 2

1 large fennel bulb,
  quartered and stems
  removed
1 tablespoon extra-virgin
  olive oil
2 tablespoons grated
  Parmesan cheese

1. Boil or steam the quartered fennel until tender; toss in extra-virgin olive oil.

2. Roast for 10 minutes at 400°F; sprinkle with Parmesan cheese, and roast for 2 additional minutes.

Asparagus in Gorgonzola Sauce

Serves 2

10 asparagus spears
Gorgonzola Sauce (page
  249)

1. Steam the asparagus spears until tender, around 10 minutes.

2. Top with Gorgonzola Sauce.

Creamy Cucumber Salad

Serves 2

½ cup plain almond or
   coconut yogurt

1 green onion, chopped

1 tablespoon sliced red
   onion

Black pepper to taste

1 tablespoon fresh dill,
   chopped, or ½ teaspoon
   dried

1 clove garlic, minced

½ cup cucumber, thinly
   sliced

1. Combine yogurt with green onion, red onion, pepper,
   dill, and garlic.

2. Add cucumbers and toss until evenly coated.

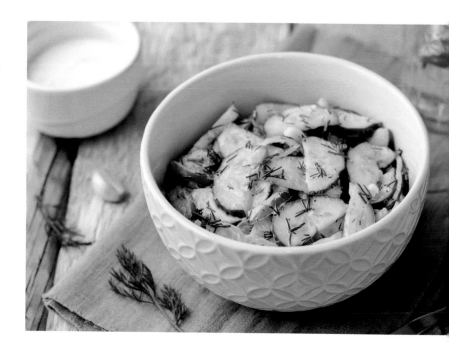

Zucchini Chips

Serves 4

2 medium zucchini
1 tablespoon oil
Salt, to taste
Your favorite seasonings,
   to taste (optional)

1. Preheat oven to 200°F.

2. Line 2 baking sheets with parchment paper.

3. Cut the zucchini into ⅛-inch slices (a mandolin works well).

4. Toss the zucchini slices in oil, salt, and your favorite seasonings.

5. Place the slices side by side (they can touch but not overlap) and bake for about 2½ hours, rotating the pans halfway through.

6. The chips are done when they are golden and just starting to get crispy. Allow them to cool in the oven with the heat off and the door propped slightly open.

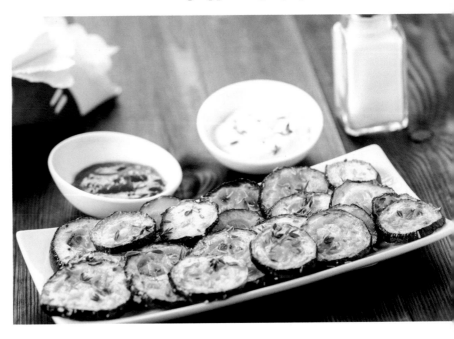

Dressings and Sauces

Creamy Alfredo Sauce

Serves 4

⅓ cup butter

2 cloves garlic, pressed

4 ounces cream cheese, cubed

1 cup half-and-half

½ cup grated Parmesan cheese

½ teaspoon dried oregano

½ teaspoon salt

½ teaspoon black pepper

1. In a medium saucepan, melt the butter over medium heat. Add the garlic and thoroughly combine.

2. Add the cream cheese and whisk constantly until the cheese is melted. Slowly pour in the half-and-half and whisk continuously until smooth.

3. Gradually add the grated Parmesan, while whisking until combined.

4. Add the oregano, salt, and pepper, and stir. Continue to simmer for 1 to 2 minutes, but do not let the sauce boil. Add more salt and pepper, to taste, if desired.

5. Remove from the heat and serve, or refrigerate in airtight containers for up to 5 days.

Low-Sugar Pizza Sauce

Makes 1 Cup

1 (5.5-ounce) can organic tomato paste

1 tablespoon dried oregano

2 teaspoons dried basil

1½ teaspoons garlic powder

1 teaspoon onion powder

¼ teaspoon salt

1 pinch ground pepper

½–1 cup water

1. Whisk together all ingredients except water.

2. Stir in water until desired consistency is reached.

3. Use immediately or refrigerate in an airtight container.

Ranch Dressing

Makes 2 Cups

1 cup mayonnaise
½ cup sour cream
2 teaspoons lemon juice
1 teaspoon dried dill
1 teaspoon dried chives
½ teaspoon garlic powder
½ teaspoon salt
½ teaspoon black pepper
¼ cup unsweetened
    almond milk

1. Whisk all ingredients (except almond milk) until thoroughly combined.

2. Gradually whisk in the almond milk until the desired consistency has been reached.

3. Refrigerate for at least 1 hour and up to 10 days.

Broccoli Picnic Salad Dressing

Makes 1 Cup

⅔ cup mayonnaise
3 tablespoons apple cider
    vinegar
1 tablespoon Dijon mustard
Salt and pepper, to taste

1. In a medium bowl, combine all ingredients.

2. Toss with your broccoli salad immediately or store in an airtight container for up to 10 days.

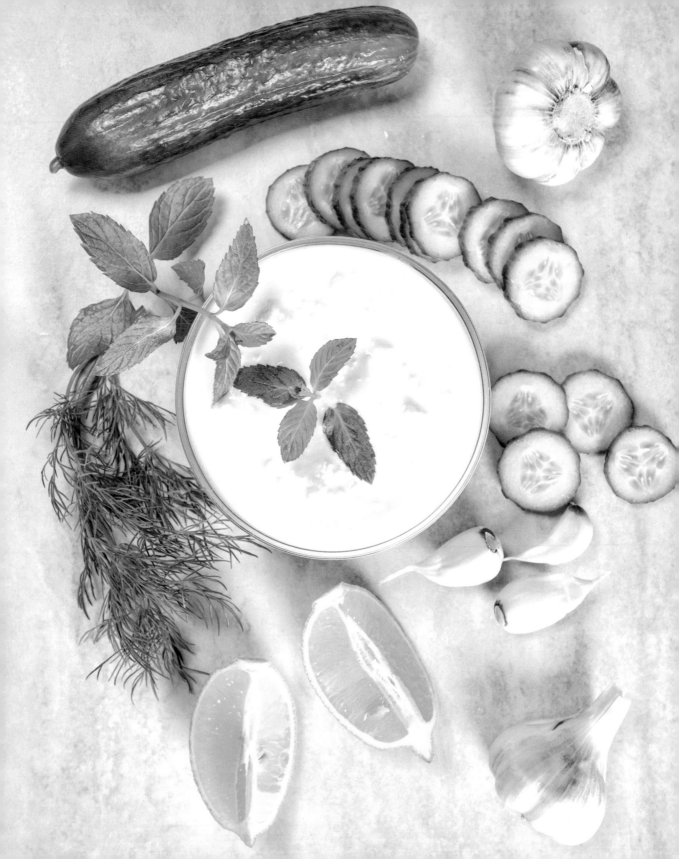

Tzatziki Dipping Sauce

Makes 1½ Cups

1 cup Greek whole milk
  yogurt
1 small cucumber, diced
2 cloves garlic, minced
2 tablespoons fresh lemon
  juice
2 tablespoons fresh dill,
  chopped
1 tablespoon fresh mint,
  finely chopped
Salt and pepper to taste
  (optional)

1. In a medium mixing bowl combine all ingredients.

2. Store an in airtight container and refrigerate for up to 7 days.

Gorgonzola Sauce

Makes 1 Cup

2 tablespoons butter
1 clove garlic, minced
⅓ cup crumbled
  Gorgonzola cheese
¼ cup grated Parmesan
  cheese
¼ cup heavy whipping
  cream
1 teaspoon onion powder
Salt and pepper, to taste

1. In small saucepan over low heat, combine the butter and garlic.

2. When the butter is melted, add the remaining the ingredients, stir, and raise the heat to medium-high.

3. Allow the sauce to come to a simmer and continue to stir for 3 to 5 minutes, allowing it to reduce until the desired consistency is achieved.

Avocado Oil Mayonnaise

Makes 1¼ Cups

1 large egg, at room
 temperature

1 teaspoon Dijon mustard

2 teaspoons apple cider
 vinegar

¼ teaspoon salt

1 cup avocado oil

1. Crack the egg in a medium bowl and place all other ingredients on top.

2. Using a hand mixer, blend on medium-high speed until a mayonnaise texture forms. Alternatively, you could combine all ingredients in a tall jar and use an immersion blender.

3. Place in an airtight container and store in the refrigerator for up to 2 weeks.

Dairy-Free Cashew Cheese Sauce

Makes 2 Cups

1½ cups raw cashew pieces

¼ cup nutritional yeast
 flakes

1 teaspoon salt

¼ teaspoon garlic powder

¾ cup water

3 tablespoons freshly
 squeezed lemon

1. In a food processor or blender, process the cashews into a fine powder, adding a drizzle of water if needed.

2. Add nutritional yeast, salt, and garlic powder, and process to combine.

3. Add lemon juice and water, and process until smooth.

Easy Caesar Dressing

Makes 1½ Cups

¾ cup mayonnaise
⅓ cup grated Parmesan
   cheese
2 cloves garlic, pressed
1 teaspoon anchovy paste
1 teaspoon lemon juice
½ teaspoon Dijon mustard
Salt and pepper, to taste

1. Place all ingredients in a medium-sized bowl and mix thoroughly combine.

2. Serve immediately or store in an airtight container in the refrigerator for up to 1 week.

Smooth Tomato and Goat Cheese

Makes 1 Cup

¼ cup crumbled goat
   cheese
2 tablespoons white wine
   vinegar
¼ cup extra-virgin olive oil
2 plum tomatoes, seeded
   and chopped
½ teaspoon salt
Freshly ground pepper, to
   taste
1 tablespoon chopped fresh
   tarragon (optional)

1. Blend all ingredients together until mixture is creamy and smooth (can be refrigerated for up to 3 days).

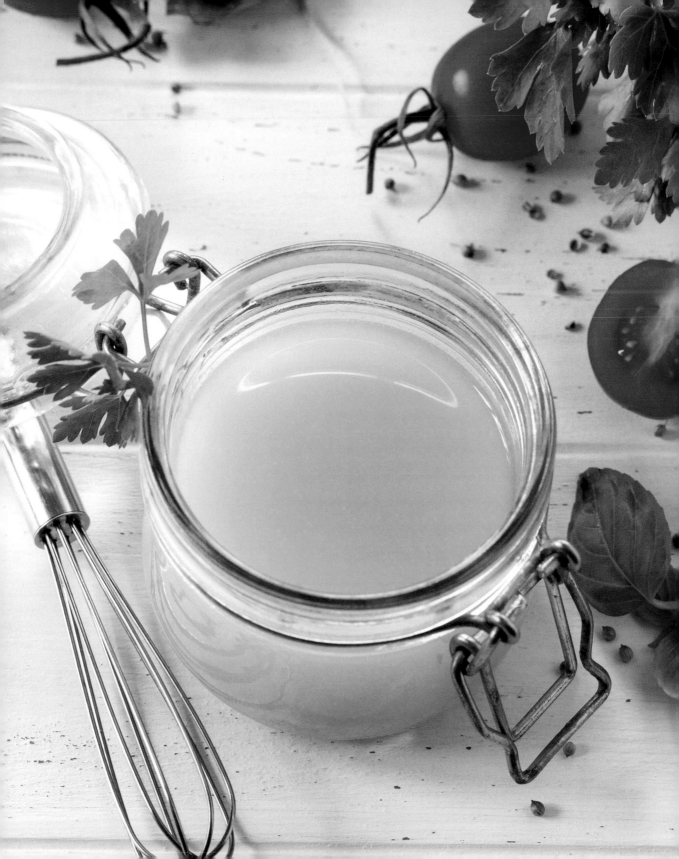

Lemon Vinaigrette

Makes 1 Cup

¼ cup red wine vinegar
2 tablespoons Dijon
    mustard
1 clove garlic, minced
1 teaspoon dried oregano
¼ teaspoon ground black
    pepper
½ cup olive oil
2 tablespoons fresh lemon
    juice

1. Whisk red wine vinegar, mustard, garlic, oregano, and black pepper in a small bowl until blended.

2. Drizzle in oil, whisking until blended.

3. Beat lemon juice into the mixture.

Green Pesto

Makes 2 Cups

1½ cups packed fresh basil
    leaves
¼ teaspoon freshly ground
    black pepper
¼ cup freshly grated
    Parmigiano-Reggiano
    (optional)
2 tablespoons pine nuts or
    walnuts
1 teaspoon minced garlic
½ cup extra-virgin olive oil

1. Using a food processor or blender, combine the basil and pepper and process/blend for a few seconds until the basil is chopped.

2. Add the cheese, pine nuts, and garlic, and while the processor is running, add the oil in a thin, steady stream until you have reached a smooth consistency.

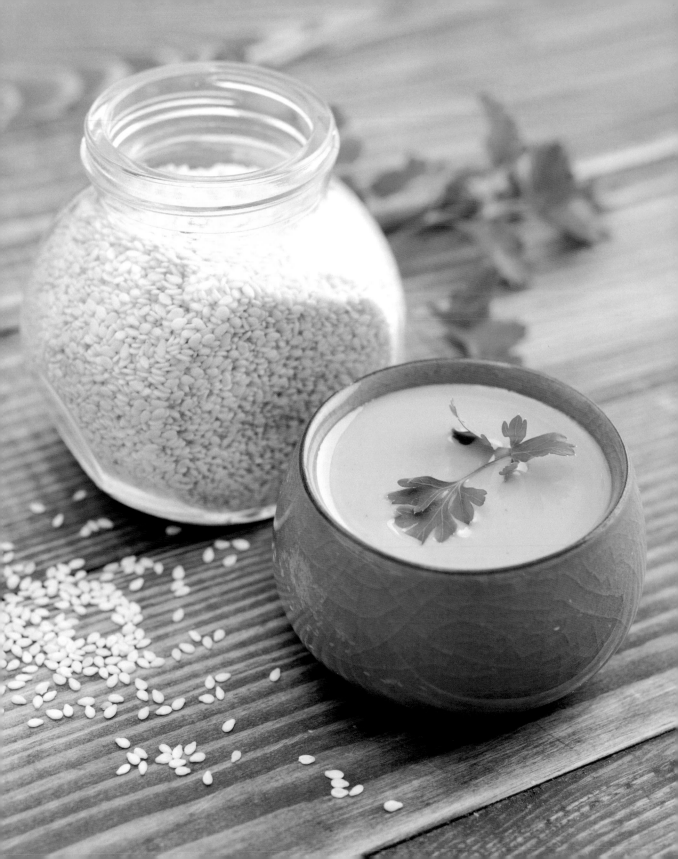

Creamy Tahini-Lemon Dressing

Makes 1 Cup

½ cup tahini
2 cloves garlic, minced
4 tablespoons fresh lemon
   juice
1 tablespoon extra-virgin
   olive oil
⅓ cup water
Salt and pepper, to taste

1. Thoroughly combine all ingredients; add more water if needed until desired consistency is reached.

2. Store in the refrigerator in an airtight container for up to 7 days.

Horseradish Cream Sauce

Makes 1¼ Cups

1 cup Greek yogurt
¼ cup grated fresh
   horseradish
1 tablespoon Dijon mustard
1 teaspoon white wine
   vinegar
¼ teaspoon freshly ground
   black pepper

1. Place all of the ingredients into a medium mixing bowl and whisk until the mixture is smooth and creamy.

2. Refrigerate for at least 4 hours to allow flavors to meld.

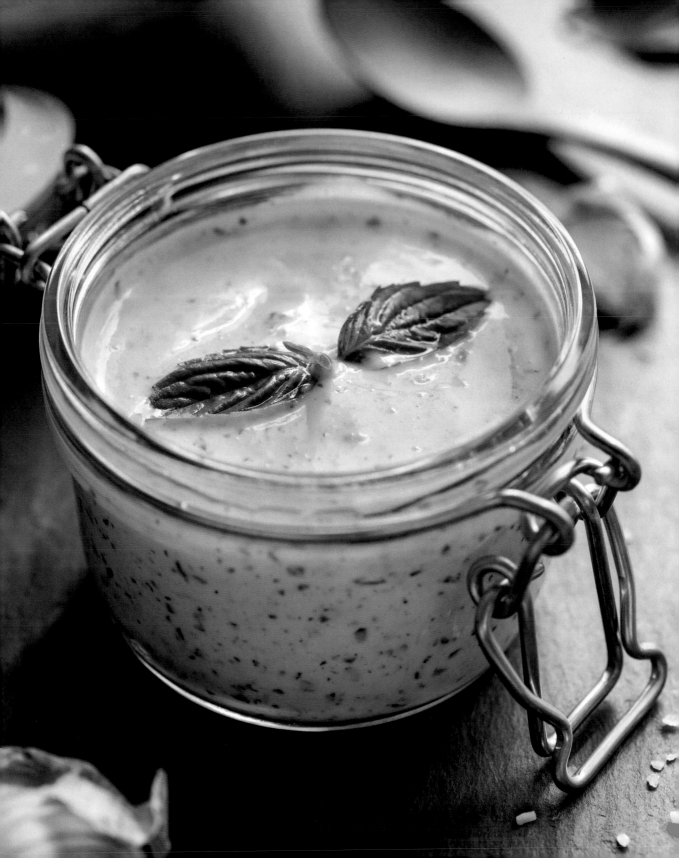

Creamy Cucumber Vinaigrette

Makes about 1 Cup

1 small cucumber, peeled, seeded, and chopped

¼ cup extra-virgin olive oil

2 tablespoons red wine vinegar

2 tablespoons chopped fresh chives

2 tablespoons chopped fresh parsley

2 tablespoons Greek yogurt

1 teaspoon prepared horseradish (optional)

1. Blend all ingredients together until mixture is creamy and smooth.

White Wine Sauce

Makes 1 Cup

½ cup chicken broth

¼ cup white wine

Juice of ½ lemon

1 tablespoon minced shallot

1 clove garlic, minced

1 tablespoon butter

1 tablespoon extra-virgin olive oil

Black pepper, to taste

1. Combine all ingredients in pan and use as a simmer sauce.

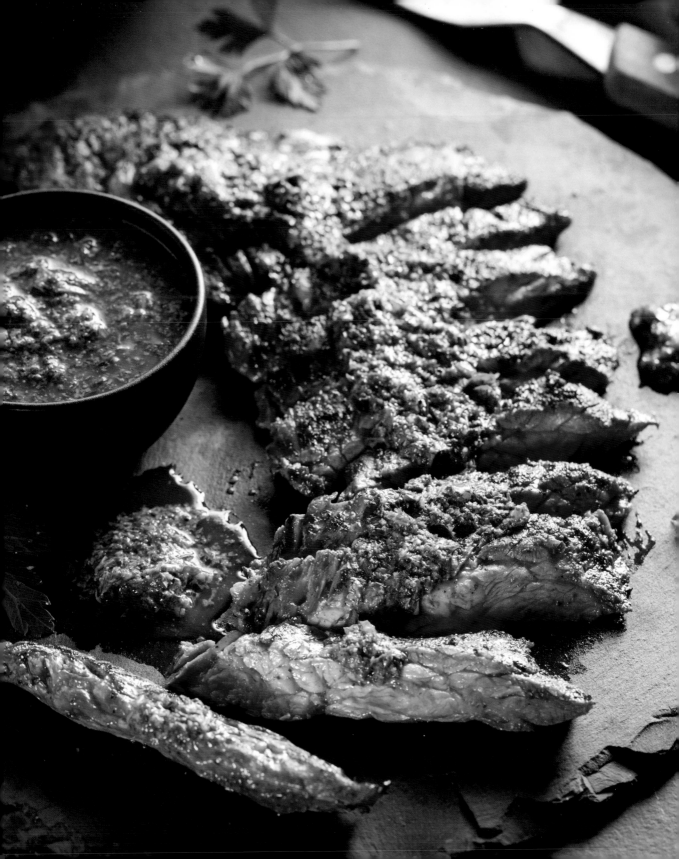

Chimichurri Sauce

Makes 1 Cup

1 bunch parsley, finely
chopped

1 bunch cilantro, finely
chopped

3 tablespoons capers, finely
chopped

2 cloves garlic, minced

1½ tablespoons red wine
vinegar

½ teaspoon red pepper
flakes

½ teaspoon ground black
pepper

½ cup extra-virgin olive oil

1. Put the parsley, cilantro, capers, and garlic in a medium
mixing bowl and toss to combine.

2. Add the vinegar, red and black pepper, and stir.

3. Pour in the olive oil and mix until well combined; let sit
for 30 minutes so that the flavors blend.

About the Authors

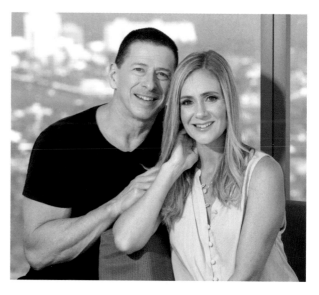

Aimee Aristotelous is the author of *Almost Keto*, *The 30-Day Keto Plan*, and *The Whole Pregnancy*, and is a certified nutritionist, specializing in ketogenic and gluten-free nutrition, as well as prenatal dietetics. Aristotelous is a contributor for a variety of publications including *Health* magazine, *People*, *Huffpost*, *Parade*, Well+Good, *INSIDER*, Motherly, *Simply Gluten Free*, Yahoo!, Consumer Health Digest, National Celiac Association, and *Delight Gluten-Free*. She has appeared on the morning show in Los Angeles, as a regular speaker for the nationwide Nourished Festival, and has been the exclusive nutritionist for NBC affiliate KSEE 24 News in California, appearing in more than fifty nutrition and cooking segments. Aimee has nine years of nutrition consulting experience and has helped over three thousand people lose weight and get healthy!

Aimee's interest in nutrition began as she struggled with her own high cholesterol and weight gain after taking a sedentary office job in her twenties, once her athletic career came to an end. She furthered her nutrition education in the ketogenic and gluten-free realms after applying those dietary lifestyles to resolve her bad cholesterol, weight gain, and other dietary-related ailments such as migraine headaches. In addition to her Nutrition and Wellness certification through American Fitness Professionals and Associates, Aimee has a bachelor's degree in business/marketing from California State University, Long

Beach. A California native, she currently resides in Fort Lauderdale, Florida, with her husband, Richard, and son, Alex, and enjoys the beach, cooking, and traveling.

Richard Oliva, co-author of *Almost Keto* and *The 30-Day Keto Plan*, is a certified nutritionist who specializes in ketogenic, gluten-free, and sports nutrition. He is a third-degree black belt in judo who has competed internationally and won state, national, and international titles. Oliva has conducted numerous nutrition seminars for colleges, health clubs, and medical practices, and has appeared in numerous nutrition and cooking segments on NBC affiliate KSEE 24 News in California. He loves to share his lifetime passion for both nutrition and judo and has helped thousands of people learn how to eat better and improve their health and fitness.

Richard began studying nutrition at about the same time that he started learning judo in the mid-1970s, when he was in high school. He became a passionate student of nutrition after one of his coworkers at the grocery store where he worked told him, "You know, you're killing yourself!" as Richard was eating a donut and drinking a soda during his break. That comment launched him on a mission to learn everything he could about nutrition and health.

Richard earned his Nutrition and Wellness certification through American Fitness Professionals and Associates. He also has a Bachelor of Science degree in geology from Kent State University. An Ohio native, he currently resides in Fort Lauderdale, Florida, with Aimee and Alex. Richard still enjoys practicing judo as well as weight training, cooking, and traveling.

References

Avena, N., P. Rada, and B. Hoebel. "Evidence for Sugar Addiction: Behavioral and Neurochemical Effects of Intermittent, Excessive Sugar Intake." NCBI. Neuroscience and Biobehavioral Reviews, January 2008. https://www.ncbi.nlm.nih.gov/pmc/articles/PMC2235907/.

Calder PC; "Marine Omega-3 Fatty Acids and Inflammatory Processes: Effects, Mechanisms and Clinical Relevance," NCBI. April 2015, https://pubmed.ncbi.nlm.nih.gov/25149823/.

Callegaro, D., and J. Tirapegui. "[Comparison of the Nutritional Value between Brown Rice and White Rice]." NCBI. October/November 1996. Accessed April 14, 2019. https://www.ncbi.nlm.nih.gov/pubmed/9302338.

Chinwong, S., D. Chinwong, and A. Mangklabruks. "Daily Consumption of Virgin Coconut Oil Increases High-Density Lipoprotein Cholesterol Levels in Healthy Volunteers: A Randomized Crossover Trial." NCBI. December 14, 2017. Accessed May 19, 2019. https://www.ncbi.nlm.nih.gov/pmc/articles/PMC5745680/.

Damle, S. G. "Smart Sugar? The Sugar Conspiracy." NCBI. July 24, 2017. Accessed March 7, 2019. https://www.ncbi.nlm.nih.gov/pmc/articles/PMC5551319/.

Dewan, Shalini Shahani. "Global Markets for Sugars and Sweeteners in Processed Foods and Beverages." Global Sugars and Sweeteners Market: Size, Share & Industry Report. BCC Research, 2015. https://www.bccresearch.com/market-research/food-and-beverage/sugar-sweeteners-processed-food-beverages-global-markets-report.html.

"Diet Review: Ketogenic Diet for Weight Loss." The Nutrition Source, May 22, 2019. https://www.hsph.harvard.edu/nutritionsource/healthy-weight/diet-reviews/ketogenic-diet/.

Feskanich et al., "Milk, dietary calcium, and bone fractures in women: a 12-year prospective study.," NCBI, June 1997, accessed September 11, 2017, https://www.ncbi.nlm.nih.gov/pmc/articles/PMC1380936/.

Finucane, O. M. et al.; "Monounsaturated Fatty Acid-Enriched High-Fat Diets Impede Adipose NLRP3 Inflammasome-Mediated IL-1β Secretion and Insulin Resistance despite Obesity," June 2015, https://pubmed.ncbi.nlm.nih.gov/25626736/.

Garg, A; "High-Monounsaturated-Fat Diets for Patients with Diabetes Mellitus: a Meta-Analysis," March 1998, https://pubmed.ncbi.nlm.nih.gov/9497173/.

Gearing, M., and S. McArdel, "Natural and Added Sugars: Two Sides of the Same Coin," October 5, 2015. https://sitn.hms.harvard.edu/flash/2015/natural-and-added-sugars-two-sides-of-the-same-coin/

Gostin, Lawrence O. ""Big Food" Is Making America Sick." NCBI. September 13, 2013. Accessed March 7, 2019. https://www.ncbi.nlm.nih.gov/pmc/articles/PMC5020160/

Hormones in Dairy Foods and Their Impact on Public Health - A Narrative Review Article, June 2015, accessed September 10, 2017, https://www.ncbi.nlm.nih.gov/pmc/articles/PMC4524299/.

Kaats, G. R., D. Bagchi, and H. G. Preuss. "Konjac Glucomannan Dietary Supplementation Causes Significant Fat Loss in Compliant Overweight Adults." NCBI. October 22, 2015. Accessed May 20, 2019. https://www.ncbi.nlm.nih.gov/pubmed/26492494.

Kabara, J., D. Swieczkowski, A. Conley, and J. Truant. "Fatty Acids and Derivatives as Antimicrobial Agents." NCBI. July 1972. Accessed May 19, 2019. https://www.ncbi.nlm.nih.gov/pmc/articles/PMC444260/.

Koller, V. J., M. Furhacker, A. Nersesyan, M. Misik, M. Eisenbauer, and S. Knasmueller. "Cytotoxic and DNA-damaging Properties of Glyphosate and Roundup in Human-derived Buccal Epithelial Cells." NCBI. May 2012. Accessed May 11, 2019. https://www.ncbi.nlm.nih.gov/pubmed/22331240.

Malekinejad, A., and H. Rezabakhsh. "Hormones in Dairy Foods and Their Impact on Public Health—A Narrative Review Article." Iranian Journal of Public Health. U.S. National Library of Medicine, June 2015. https://pubmed.ncbi.nlm.nih.gov/26258087/.

Maruyama, Kazumi, T. Oshima, and K. Ohyama, "Exposure to exogenous estrogen through intake of commercial milk produced from pregnant cows." NCBI, February 2010, accessed September 20, 2017, https://pubmed.ncbi.nlm.nih.gov/19496976/.

McNamara, Donald. "The Fifty Year Rehabilitation of the Egg." NCBI. October 2015. Accessed April 27, 2019. https://www.ncbi.nlm.nih.gov/pmc/articles/PMC4632449/.

Michaëlsson, K. et al., "Milk intake and risk of mortality and fractures in women and men: cohort studies." NCBI, October 28, 2014, accessed September 20, 2017, https://www.ncbi.nlm.nih.gov/pubmed/25352269.

Missimer, A., D. DiMarco, C. Andersen, A. Murillo, M. Vergara-Jiminez, and M. Fernandez. "Consuming Two Eggs per Day, as Compared to an Oatmeal Breakfast, Decreases Plasma Ghrelin While Maintaining the LDL/HDL Ratio." NCBI. February 01, 2017. Accessed April 27, 2019. https://www.ncbi.nlm.nih.gov/pmc/articles/PMC5331520/.

Mozaffarian, Dariush, Tao Hao, Eric Rimm, Walter Willett, and Frank Hu. "Changes in Diet and Lifestyle and Long-Term Weight Gain in Women and Men." *The New England Journal of Medicine*. June 29, 2011. Accessed April 14, 2019. https://www.nejm.org/doi/full/10.1056/NEJMoa1014296.

Mumme, K., and W. Stonehouse. "Effects of Medium-chain Triglycerides on Weight Loss and Body Composition: A Meta-analysis of Randomized Controlled Trials." NCBI. February 2015. Accessed May 19, 2019. https://www.ncbi.nlm.nih.gov/pubmed/25636220.

Nestle, M. "Food Lobbies, the Food Pyramid, and U.S. Nutrition Policy." NCBI. July 1, 1993. Accessed February 16, 2019. https://www.ncbi.nlm.nih.gov/pubmed/8375951.

Ng, S. W., M. M. Slining, and B. M. Popkin. (2012). Use of caloric and noncaloric sweeteners in US consumer packaged foods, 2005–2009. *Journal of the Academy of Nutrition and Dietetics*, 112(11), 1828–1834. e1821-1826.

Niaz, K., E. Zaplatic, and J. Spoor. "Extensive Use of Monosodium Glutamate: A Threat to Public Health?" NCBI. March 19, 2018. Accessed May 11, 2019. https://www.ncbi.nlm.nih.gov/pmc/articles/PMC5938543/.

Paoli, Antonio. "Ketogenic Diet for Obesity: Friend or Foe?" NCBI. February 01, 2014. Accessed March 23, 2019. https://www.ncbi.nlm.nih.gov/pmc/articles/PMC3945587/.

C. S. Pase et al., "Influence of perinatal trans fat on behavioral responses and brain oxidative status of adolescent rats acutely exposed to stress.," NCBI, September 05, 2013, accessed September 02, 2017, https://www.ncbi.nlm.nih.gov/pubmed/23742847.

Price, Sterling. "Average Household Cost of Food," June 19, 2020. https://www.valuepenguin.com/how-much-we-spend-food.

Samsel, A., and S. Seneff. "Glyphosate, Pathways to Modern Diseases II: Celiac Sprue and Gluten Intolerance." NCBI. December 2013. Accessed May 11, 2019. https://www.ncbi.nlm.nih.gov/pmc/articles/PMC3945755/.

Santarelli, RL, F. Pierre, and D. Corpet. "Processed Meat and Colorectal Cancer: A Review of Epidemiologic and Experimental Evidence." NCBI. March 25, 2008. Accessed April 14, 2019. https://www.ncbi.nlm.nih.gov/pmc/articles/PMC2661797/.

Soffritti, M., M. Padovani, E. Tibalidi, L. Falcioni, F. Manservisi, and F. Belpoggi. "The Carcinogenic Effects of Aspartame: The Urgent Need for Regulatory Re-evaluation." NCBI. April 2014. Accessed April 14, 2019. https://www.ncbi.nlm.nih.gov/pubmed/24436139.

Spero, David, and Bsn. "Is Milk Bad for You? Diabetes and Milk - Diabetes Self." Management. Diabetes Self Management, June 20, 2017. https://www.diabetesselfmanagement.com/blog/is-milk-bad-for-you-diabetes-and-milk/.

Mary-Catherine Stockman et al., "Intermittent Fasting: Is the Wait Worth the Weight?" June 2018, https://www.ncbi.nlm.nih.gov/pmc/articles/PMC5959807/.

"Sugar & The Diet." The Sugar Association. Accessed March 5, 2020. https://www.sugar.org/diet/.

Swithers, S. "Artificial sweeteners produce the counterintuitive effect of inducing metabolic derangements," NCBI, September 2013, accessed September 24, 2017, https://www.ncbi.nlm.nih.gov/pmc/articles/PMC3772345/.

Zhang, G., A. Pan, G. Zhong, Z. Yu, H. Wu, X. Chen, L. Tang, Y. Feng, H. Zhou, H. Li, B. Hong, W. C. Willett, V. S. Malik, D. Spiegelman, F. B. Hu, and X. Lin. "Substituting White Rice with Brown Rice for 16 Weeks Does Not Substantially Affect Metabolic Risk Factors in Middle-aged Chinese Men and Women with Diabetes or a High Risk for Diabetes." NCBI. September 01, 2011. Accessed April 14, 2019. https://pubmed.ncbi.nlm.nih.gov/21795429/.

Conversion Charts

Metric and Imperial Conversions
(These conversions are rounded for convenience)

Ingredient	Cups/ Tablespoons/ Teaspoons	Ounces	Grams/Milliliters
Butter	1 cup/ 16 tablespoons/ 2 sticks	8 ounces	230 grams
Cheese, shredded	1 cup	4 ounces	110 grams
Cream cheese	1 tablespoon	0.5 ounce	14.5 grams
Fruit, dried	1 cup	4 ounces	120 grams
Fruits or veggies, chopped	1 cup	5 to 7 ounces	145 to 200 grams
Fruits or veggies, pureed	1 cup	8.5 ounces	245 grams
Liquids: cream, milk, water, or juice	1 cup	8 fluid ounces	240 milliliters
Salt	1 teaspoon	0.2 ounce	6 grams
Spices: cinnamon, cloves, ginger, or nutmeg (ground)	1 teaspoon	0.2 ounce	5 milliliters
Vanilla extract	1 teaspoon	0.2 ounce	4 grams

Oven Temperatures

Fahrenheit	Celsius	Gas Mark
225°	110°	¼
250°	120°	½
275°	140°	1
300°	150°	2
325°	160°	3
350°	180°	4
375°	190°	5
400°	200°	6
425°	220°	7
450°	230°	8

Index